December 2001

To Jenny,

Lots of love,

Marissa

Listen to the Lighten Up audio book.
Published by Random House and
available from all good bookshops.

ISBN 1856865452

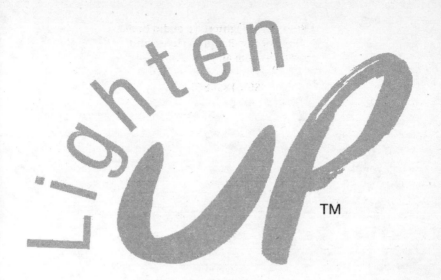

Lighten up ™

Pete Cohen
and
Judith Verity

Century. London

Published by Century in 2001

3 5 7 9 10 8 6 4 2

First published in the United Kingdom in 2001 by Century

Random House Group Limited
20 Vauxhall Bridge Road, London SW1V 2SA

Random House Australia (Pty) Limited
20 Alfred Street, Milsons Point, Sydney,
New South Wales 2061, Australia

Random House New Zealand Limited
18 Poland Road, Glenfield
Auckland 10, New Zealand

Random House (Pty) Limited
Endulini, 5a Jubilee Road, Parktown 2193,
South Africa

Random House Group Limited Reg. No. 954009

A CIP catalogue record for this book is available
from the British Library

Papers used by Random House are natural, recyclable products made from wood grown in sustainable forests. The manufacturing processes conform to the environmental regulations of the country of origin

ISBN 0 7126 7034 3

Design & make up by Roger Walker

Printed and bound in Great Britain by
Bookmarque Ltd, Croydon, Surrey

To

Jane Carter
Wendy Chappell
Sally Coleman
Jo Hardy
Caroline Harper
Clare McCaffrey
Loraine Prokopiou
Lindsey Sills & Kerry Larcher
Sarah Tay
Jonathan Zneimer

the first Lighten Up presenters.

CONTENTS

Part Three

FOREWORD

I joined the Lighten Up team in February 2000 because I was really impressed by their approach to helping people become slimmer. My own experience has taught me that motivation is the key to success – not only in sport but in everything else in life - and slimming is no exception. What I love about Lighten Up is that it puts motivation back into the eating and exercise equation, and the amazing success rate speaks for itself.

If you lead a busy life – and especially if you have family responsibilities as well – it's all too easy to neglect your own health and well-being. But, in the long run, you'll achieve more at work and set a better example to your children if you look after yourself. The Lighten Up programme will help you take better care of yourself and start believing in that image of a slimmer, fitter, healthier you.

This book takes you, step-by-step and day-by-day, through the highly successful eight week slimming course, and it gives you all the information you need about nutrition and exercise as well. You will learn how to eat when you're hungry (instead of when you're tired and stressed), how to choose the kinds of food your body really needs, how to enjoy a more active lifestyle, and how to be a slimmer, happier person.

It's definitely one of those books that will change your life – and, as you read it, you find that making those changes can be a lot of fun.

Good luck!

Sally Gunnell

Sally Gunnell

INTRODUCTION

Welcome to the revolutionary Lighten Up eight-week slimming programme! Week by week and step by step, it will guide you towards a slimmer, fitter, healthier you. It's easy to follow and a lot of fun, providing simple, straightforward advice on exercise and nutrition, and enabling you to make your own lifestyle changes.

But how is Lighten Up different?

Lighten Up is different because it is the first slimming programme to put *you* in control of your eating habits and free you from the dieting trap so that you can start feeling better about yourself and enjoying a healthier, happier lifestyle. As your self-image becomes stronger and more positive you will find you have more energy and confidence – and you will look great!

My name is Pete Cohen and I started Lighten Up about ten years ago when I realised that many of the people who came to me for fitness training were also fighting a constant battle to control their weight. I discovered what most people who've tried to lose weight know already – that dieting alone doesn't work and can even be dangerous. And I also found my clients didn't stick with rigorous exercise programmes. The big breakthrough came when I realised that the motivational techniques I used to help athletes in training worked just as well for slimmers, and that's what makes Lighten Up unique.

Several years ago I met Judith Verity and, together, we decided to write this book about the Lighten Up programme. It's taken a while to put Lighten Up into words and this is the first time that the entire programme has been available in one book, together with lots of advice on exercise and nutrition. We've even included some of our favourite recipes at the back. During the time that Judith and I have been working together, the Lighten Up message has been spreading fast. We now have eight-week courses running nationwide and a great support team of nutritionists, fitness experts and presenters led by Sally Gunnell who is now our chief spokesperson.

This means that we are able to follow up and offer support to everyone who reads about us or comes on one of our courses. In fact some of the feedback we've received from Lighten Uppers over the years has gone into this book. Of course, it also contains a lot of my own personal experience from back in the early days, and Judith and I both hope that you'll have fun reading it, as well as getting all the help you need.

We call Lighten Up 'slimming from the head down', so reading about it and thinking about it for yourself is a very good place to start. The Lighten Up programme has proved that just *trying* to diet, or trying to 'be good', isn't enough. Unless you really change the way you feel about eating – and bear in mind here that most people in this country have a rather complicated relationship with food – you'll never truly lose weight for good. You might be *temporarily* thinner, but the chances are it won't make you happy.

Part Two of the book is the eight-week course that will help you become slimmer and stay slimmer permanently. Sounds appealing, doesn't it? And it really does work, but although you'll probably want to get started straight away, please do read Part One first. It won't take long and it will help you to get the most out of the eight-week course in Part Two. Relax and give yourself the time you need. Remember, these are lifetime changes you're about to make.

So, good luck from all of us at Lighten Up. If this is the first slimming book you've ever bought, then all we can say is good choice! *And if it's not your first time – be prepared for this one to be different.*

PART

CHAPTER ONE

WHAT HAVE YOU GOT TO LOSE?

> *How many times have you tried to lose weight?*
> *And how important is it to succeed?*

THE BIG ISSUE

One of the first news items of the new millennium was the headline that, for the first time, the number of starving people in the world is roughly equal to the number of people who are clinically obese. This shocking news seems to be the ultimate proof that, for a lot of human beings, food is a problem. If you don't get enough food you die. And if you get too much food, you die a bit slower.

Maybe this is why slimming has never been taken very seriously – after all, when people in underdeveloped countries are starving it seems a bit petty to complain about having too much food. And perhaps because slimming's been considered such a trivial topic, nobody's questioned some of the rubbish that's been written about it over the past fifty years or so.

But telling your children to finish their dinner because their brothers and sisters in the Third World are undernourished isn't going to change the balance. All it's likely to achieve is yet another generation of plate emptiers who end up overweight because they are eating for the wrong reasons.

Maybe, if we could teach our children not to take food for granted, the adults of the future might have a little more respect for the balance between their own needs and the needs of others. But, realistically, none of this is going to have any effect on obesity, which is becoming more of an issue every day while the secondary problem of eating disorders is affecting more and more young people. Obesity and eating disorders, like famine are potentially fatal conditions.

The Brits are getting bigger

The 1985 report by the US National Institute of Health concluded that obesity should be viewed as a disease. Fifteen years on, most authorities agree that obesity, like smoking, is a major trigger for heart problems – the biggest cause of death in the UK. And heart disease isn't the only risk factor: the NHS was recently reported to be spending £1.73 billion a year on treating overweight people suffering from conditions directly related to their weight such as heart disease, strokes and cancer. Think *what else £1.73 billion could buy for our overstretched Health Service!*

You probably won't be terribly surprised to hear that the Americans are the world's fattest nation – according to the World Health Organisation 59 per cent of US males and 49 per cent of US women are obese – but Britain is one of the fattest nations in Europe. It's estimated that the *entire* US population will be overweight by 2030 and it seems that (according to the NPD market research company which specialises in tracking eating habits) the main reason Americans are getting fatter is simply that health is bottom of their list of priorities. Could this be true for us too?

In July 2000 the Medical Research Council sent a report to all British MPs warning that 50 per cent of adults in the UK are overweight and that government targets for reducing cancer and heart disease won't be met unless there's a national effort to cut obesity. According to the report, 'There is a pressing need to recognise that obesity and overweight place an enormous strain on our health and on NHS resources . . . Obesity is a missing link in the chain of health problems.'

This is serious stuff. It is quite clear that obesity and eating disorders are serious health risks. They are getting out of control. So surely there must be more to slimming than vanity or fashion, mustn't there? Slimming is important, and it's important on a global scale. But concern about the future of humanity isn't going to help *you* lose weight, so what you need to decide is: how important is slimming to you?

When I walk into a Lighten Up workshop and look at the people sitting in the seats in front of me, I often feel I'm much more motivated about them being slimmer and healthier than they are themselves. The number of reasons people find for not losing weight is amazing, but then the fact that they've been overweight or worrying about it for so long is pretty amazing too.

So I'm going to ask you the question I always like to ask up front: *How much do you really want to be slimmer?*

If you don't have a go, you'll never know

You've bought the book, and that's a start. But lots of people buy books and some rather alarming research tells us that 90 per cent of them don't get past the first chapter. So your first challenge is easy: I dare you to read on. Let your mind play with the ideas as you go along and if your body wants to join in it's welcome.

Never say later – Lighten Up really can work for you

If you're overweight and unfit, it's OK. If you think you've got fat genes, it's OK. If you've dieted before and the weight's always sneaked back on when you stopped concentrating, that's OK too. You've worked hard at being overweight and you're good at it. But if you've really decided to change we have some great news for you: those skills you've used to stay fat will come in just as handy for losing the weight and keeping it off. Your focus, persistence and belief in yourself will work just as well for losing weight as they did for gaining it.

You're probably not motivated enough right now to make the changes you want to make. You probably have a lot of doubts, based on your past experiences of dieting and exercising. And that's why the Lighten Up programme starts right *here*. We don't expect you suddenly, instantaneously to believe you're going to change your eating patterns, your exercise patterns, your shape, your mind and your relationship with yourself. In fact, we're going to make it easy for you by telling you to stay right where you are and read on for a while – you don't have to *do* anything yet.

All you need to change at the moment is your mind. And there's no rush on that, just keep it open.

WHAT DO I KNOW?

When I first started to run slimming workshops I was constantly being challenged by people who came up to me and said, 'You don't know what it's like to be overweight so how can you possibly help me?'

I have two answers to that:

★ I know how to be slim – and I can show you how it's done. You don't need me to show you what it's like to be overweight, you can do that already.

★ I know how to face challenges and overcome them. Whether you're worried about your weight, or you want to fix a phobia or you need to start a new career, the techniques you use are the same. My particular challenge was getting an education: I was diagnosed severely dyslexic when I was a child and all my teachers from junior school up predicted that I would never amount to anything or achieve anything academic. I was determined to prove them wrong and although I left school at sixteen with few qualifications, I now have more degrees than GCSEs.

How did I do it? Well, I suppose I was using some of the Lighten Up techniques before I even knew what they were, and the most important thing I did was to *change my beliefs*. I realised that I didn't have to accept what everybody else believed about me and, once I knew that, it was easy to create a whole new belief system of my own. The difference was that this time the beliefs were positive ones.

The other question people ask me is how I got so interested in slimming. Well although I've never done it, slimming has been part of my life ever since I can remember. Like a lot of non-dieters, I have lived with the effects of dieting on the people around me and I've always been amazed at the amount of time people spend counting calories and making themselves miserable without any obvious long-term results.

Diet is a four-letter word

My mum always told me to eat up everything on my plate so that I'd grow up to be a big strong boy. And she also told me not to use four-letter words. But she was always on a diet and I can remember watching in disbelief the bad days when the scales dictated her mood and destroyed her self-esteem.

Then, when I became a personal trainer, I realised that an awful lot of my clients – even some of the very fittest ones – were fighting a permanent battle against their weight (and against themselves). That's when I decided that this hidden agenda needed to be tackled so I started with exercise, designing wonderful workout programmes for my clients that they didn't stick to. Then I looked at it from the point of view of nutrition and drew up beautifully balanced diet sheets that they didn't stick to either. And then the penny dropped and it occurred to me that the sports psychology I used when I worked with athletes held the answer. Of course, that was over ten years ago, and Lighten Up has been developing and evolving ever since, but the starting point is always the same: how strong is your belief that you can be slim?

Exercise and eating are a vitally important part of the Lighten Up programme, but it always begins with *what's going on in your head*. Lighten Up gives you information so that you can have choices and options about what will work for you, but what makes Lighten Up different is that we will provide you with the knowledge you need to change yourself, instead of feeding you

I think I 'caught' dieting from my older sister, although it didn't really get a hold on me until I was in my twenties. At one point my father, a no-nonsense man, got hold of the bathroom scales and ripped them in two! (I think Pete would agree with that as at least a good start!)

So I watched my sister go through years of being unhappy with her weight, dieting and then putting the weight back on. Then, suddenly (it seemed) I started to notice an increase when I got on the scales myself. It was a shock and for the first time in my life I started keeping an eye on what I was eating and then began to exercise, with no great knowledge of what I should really be doing. I started to lose weight and became quite calorie conscious, while still managing to maintain my addiction to chocolate. What saved me from going too far down the obsessional route was my enjoyment of martial arts – serious training and traditional diets just don't go together. But eventually, during a period when I was injured, I came across Lighten Up and realised that this was the common sense I had been looking for.

I read as much as I could and attended one of the Lighten Up programmes. Before long I was hooked, I believed that Lighten Up was the key to freeing people from obsessive dieting and a depressing lifestyle. And, as I learned more about it, I began to notice that, although I wasn't a dieter I actually still had some unresolved issues with food. I noticed that I would eat if I was bored or fed up and I had a nice little chocolate habit hidden away. I hadn't thought too much about it, but my diet wasn't as well-balanced as it could be. I only needed to make some small changes but my eating patterns now are so much more healthy. And, yes, I do have the odd piece of chocolate and I don't beat myself up about it! In fact, I enjoy it.

Clare McCaffrey

false promises and complicated programmes that are difficult to follow. We want you to choose your own outcome and make it happen with some simple but highly effective behaviour changes.

BELIEFS

Changing negative beliefs is right at the heart of the Lighten Up programme. If you think you're fat, or unattractive, or lazy, or addicted to food, you're probably right. Right now. But you can change your mind if you want to and, if you change your mind, your body will follow.

So maybe what you really need to lose is some of those beliefs that have been holding you back. After all, the chances are you've tried to lose weight before you bought this book. And if you've tried once, you've probably tried a hundred times. What stopped you succeeding? Did you ever *really* believe it was possible? Did you ever *really* believe you would change your shape for ever?

Believe in yourself

The most important factors in successful slimming are psychological, not physical.

What's the difference between someone who manages to lose weight and someone who doesn't? Well, one person may have more of a natural tendency to hold on to fat cells than another (we'll explain about that in the next couple of chapters), but that unlucky person is just as likely to be a successful slimmer as someone who doesn't have any overweight tendencies at all.

The most obvious difference (apart from size) between someone who's lost weight and someone who hasn't will be their belief in themselves. Our behaviour depends totally on what we believe is possible for us.

A beggar stopped me recently on a street corner and I paused, because something about him was familiar. I looked again and recognised a boy I used to know at school. 'What happened to you?' I asked him.

'I didn't have a chance,' he said. 'School never did anything for me and everybody used to tell me I'd end up in trouble. Mind you,' he added, 'I never thought you were going anywhere either.'

'Maybe not,' I thought, 'but *I* did.'

Does that sound harsh? I think it's much harsher to assume that someone who's had a bad start will automatically end up at the bottom of the pile. If you take that view of things, you are going to have to accept that nobody has a choice. Even worse, you're going to have to accept that you don't have any choices either. And that includes choices about your weight.

The dining table

So, here's what you need to know about beliefs. Basically, they are like tables – they need legs to support them, otherwise they are just vague ideas that won't amount to anything. Do you really have a belief that you could be slimmer, fitter and healthier? Or is it just an idea? If it's only an idea that you like the sound of, then all you've got is the table top and you're going to have to eat off the floor.

You need some legs to support that idea and turn it into an elegant dining table, and those legs are the actions you are going to take to become slimmer. The legs might be: taking more exercise, eating when you are hungry instead of when you're stressed, choosing healthy food and following the Lighten Up programme. In fact, each week we'll be giving you more legs to support your belief so that your table will stand up, no matter how heavily you lean on it. By Week Eight you'll have a table with so many legs that it looks like a giant hairbrush. It won't matter if you kick one of them away by not exercising for a day or two, or eating too much at a party.

Knowing what to believe

Think of something you believe, something you're sure is true. Maybe you think the sun's going to come up in the morning. Maybe you think *Titanic* is your favourite film. Maybe you think toilets need cleaning. You weren't born believing any of those things. It took years of experience or repeated actions on your part to make you certain of them. In fact, some psychologists say that we have to repeat something at least twenty times before we get the hang of it. But the really interesting thing is that once we've adopted a belief, our brain will go to great lengths to validate that belief for us – even if it isn't doing us any good.

Lots of people who want to lose weight have really negative beliefs in themselves, but they weren't born thinking they were fat and unattractive. They just picked that up somewhere along the way and they can always drop it again, with a bit of help.

And a lot of people are pretty sure that losing weight is a waste of time. They've failed before (many times), they've been disappointed, so they certainly aren't going to put much heart and soul into their latest attempt. It's going to be half-hearted at best, because they're expecting failure and frustration.

So make a start. Get yourself a table top and we'll work on the legs together. Choose a belief and get used to it, because you're going to be living and breathing it for the foreseeable future. How about 'I'm getting slimmer, fitter and healthier'? It's just a suggestion, by all means choose another of your own, just make sure it's a positive one and that it's in the present tense.

Start Lightening Up

Why are there so many bizarre and complicated diet plans around? Because they fit in beautifully with the popular belief that change must be difficult. You can say to yourself 'I never thought of eating coconut and boiled eggs for every meal – no wonder I never managed to lose weight before.' You know it's crazy, but it sounds drastic enough to do the trick. You know you're going to hate every minute of it so maybe, just maybe, this one will work for you.

Well, Lighten Up is different. It's not about rules and formulas and calculations. It's about motivating yourself to make simple, comfortable changes in your life and we'll be taking you through the Eight-week Lighten Up course in Part Two of this book. Do you think a course sounds like a lot of hard work? Then why don't you think of it as a holiday instead – because you will be taking a permanent holiday from the self-limiting beliefs that stopped you losing weight in the past. And the great thing about this holiday is that we've already packed everything you need.

All you have to do is sit down and read on.

THE CHALLENGE

Go out and buy yourself a nice big fat notebook, with plenty of space in it and a cover design you like – one that makes you smile, perhaps. When you get to Chapter Nine, you will be keeping your Food Diary in it, but you can begin using it right away. Whenever you want to make a note of anything, just start a new page for each day you make an entry and put the date at the top. You'll notice as you read through the rest of Part One and start on Part Two that writing things down is quite a big part of the Lighten Up programme, and it's very important that you actually *do* it. We know it feels a bit odd to begin with, but please do try it. It might seem a bit silly, but it works – trust us.

So take ten minutes this week to sit and write down exactly why you want to be slimmer – and really think about it. Is it for the sake of your health, your relationships, your job or your self-esteem? Or is it something else?

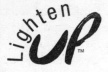

The first step to losing weight is believing you can do it.
How are you going to support that belief?

CHAPTER TWO

AN INDUSTRY FOUNDED ON FAILURE

> *How many people do you know who succeeded in losing weight –
> and didn't gain it back again?*

DIETING IS A RECIPE FOR DISASTER, NOT A SLIMMING STRATEGY

Diets involve pain and deprivation, and are inherently repetitive: you overeat, you go on a diet, it becomes unbearable therefore you overeat; you feel disgusted and so you diet again . . .

At a party I went to recently a slim and rather beautiful lady asked me, 'What's Lighten Up all about?' As soon as the words 'weight control' were out of my mouth she cut in, 'Oh, I see, it's a diet – I've just done the cabbage soup one, it was great.'

I was surprised, 'You don't need to diet, do you?'

'Well, it's a constant battle,' she said sadly.

The trouble is that as soon as you mention slimming, a neon sign saying **diet**, flashes up in most people's minds and their thinking capabilities power down. We tend to put our faith in anything that involves calculations because it looks scientific. We head for the kitchen when the clock says it's mealtime with a calorie chart in our hand instead of a recipe book. That way we feel as though we're in control.

It all started when a couple of doctors[1] at Michigan University in the 1930s came up with the theory that if we eat fewer calories than our body burns we are bound to lose weight. According to the theory, if we use 2500 calories in a day and we only eat 1500 calories then we make up the shortfall by burning 1000 calories out of our personal fat store.

And the medical profession has stuck with this method of weight control ever since. It's easy to prescribe, it's cheap, everybody can understand it, you can blame the patient for cheating if it doesn't work, and it often does work in the short term. But in spite of the fact that this theory has fuelled thousands of diets, it doesn't usually produce lasting results.

A little knowledge is a dangerous thing

The medical profession and the miracle diets are right. You can lose a lot of weight very quickly if you cut back drastically on your calorie intake. But it's not going to be either healthy, or permanent, weight loss.

Since the 1930s we've learned a lot about just how complex and delicate the balance of weight control really is. The 'calories in equals calories out' theory works for steam engines, but comparing the human body to something as crude as a steam engine is much too simplistic to be genuinely useful. Research has taught us a lot about the psychological and biochemical factors involved in weight loss. But we still have a long way to go – after all, science understands only about 5 per cent of all there is to know about how our bodies and minds actually work (in spite of the fact that the human genome is nearly complete).

It seems to us that as soon as we get part of the answer about anything, we immediately jump to the conclusion that we know it all and start drawing up lists of rules about it. Instead of staying flexible and waiting to see how much more there is to know,

1 Dr Newburgh and Dr Johnston, University of Michigan, USA, 1930.

we pitch right in and give ourselves a hard time when our rigid rules are difficult to follow and don't usually work.

So if it's a diet you want, you've come to the wrong place. A diet is just a set of rules and losing weight is both simpler and more subtle than that. The Lighten Up programme will offer you more choices and show you that you're infinitely more capable of being slim than you thought. In fact, you already have everything you need to be the way you want to be, but maybe, as we said in the last chapter, you aren't ready to believe that yet. Our aim is to unlock your confidence, your desire and your motivation to be permanently slimmer, fitter and healthier.

WHY DIETS DON'T WORK

In 1992 the National Institute of Health in the US analysed 27 pounds of documents provided by weight loss centres (why did they weigh them?) and concluded that 'there is no good evidence that any popular weight loss programme has much chance for long-term success'. But in spite of that, 25 per cent of men and 45 per cent of women are trying to lose weight at any one time according to the American Dietetic Association. Millions of people are fighting battles they can't win against bulges they can't lose.

We had an unsolicited fax the other day with the headline: LOSE TEN POUNDS IN A WEEK. If you get one of these, before you rush to pick up the phone, stop to ask yourself, 'ten pounds of what?' Because we can tell you that it won't be fat – you can't lose more than two pounds of fat in a week. Do you really want to start shedding muscle, or dehydrating?

Over the last few millennia our amazing bodies have developed an incredible system to keep us alive through periods when food is scarce – the ability to store food in the form of fat for use during the lean times. It's a wonderful system, but it's also a major problem for everyone who lives with food mountains rather than famine.

Although we have evolved past that primitive lifestyle, we still have the survival mechanism, so whenever we seriously restrict our calorie intake our bodies assume there's a food shortage and hold on to the fat we've got stored in case things get worse. But we need to stay alive so we start burning lean muscle tissue instead – and how depressing is that! Every time you go on a crash diet you are going to lose some muscle until your body adjusts itself to getting by on fewer calories. But the chances are that by the time your body has made this delicate adjustment you'll have given up on the diet, so when you start eating normally again your body is overwhelmed with the extra food and starts slapping it straight back on as fat. Your metabolism – the rate at which your body burns those calories – can remain lower than usual for weeks after you finish a diet. Your body remembers how much fat you used to have and wants to put it back quickly in case you suddenly start dieting again. Which, of course, you usually do.

Think of your body as a fireplace; the fire is your metabolism and the logs are the food. If you disappear for the day and leave the fire unattended, the chances are that when you come back to it in the evening it will be almost out. You might stoke it up with logs to get it going again, but the embers won't be hot enough to get them burning. When you look at the fireplace the next morning, you might find your logs from the night before are still lying there, a little charred, perhaps, but not burnt up. If you have a habit of going for long periods without food, your metabolism will slow right down. Perhaps you're working hard so you skip lunch, finish work late and stop for a pizza on the way home. By that time, of course, you'll be feeling pretty hungry – but don't be fooled. Your metabolism will have virtually given up by then. Eating a big meal and going straight to bed means you've got less chance of digesting that food quickly and burning it up. It's much more likely to be turned into fat and stored. If you eat small amounts regularly, you will have a better chance of using it up as you go along.

This has all been tested over and over again on laboratory rats. In a 1986 study[2] a bunch of rats were examined as they lost and gained weight, and each time they went through the cycle their metabolism got slower. By the second time around, the weight loss was half as fast and the weight was gained back *three*

2 *Physiology and Behaviour*, 1986, 38:559–64.

times as quickly. I don't understand why the researchers had to put the rats through all that. We could have told them what was going to happen – and so could hundreds of slimmers we know.

Bad news

The really bad news is that when crash dieting causes our bodies to start burning muscle in order to save the precious fat, we are making matters even worse, because lean muscles are great fat burners, so losing muscle decreases our ability to burn fat.

More bad news

When we cut back on the amount of food we eat by dieting we also cut our intake of nutrients. Unfortunately some of those nutrients, such as magnesium and the B vitamins, are essential for the reactions that burn food for energy. So just as we can't afford to lose calorie-burning muscle, we also don't want to cut back on our supply of the vitamins and minerals that trigger that fat-burning process.

Good news

The good news is that this gives us the clue to the failure factor which is built into dieting: there is a vital missing ingredient, which, of course, is exercise.

Dieting alone will never make you slim. But exercise builds muscles – which burn calories even when we aren't actually using them. However, our addiction to diets is equalled only by our addiction to not doing very much – apparently only 20–30 per cent of the population are active enough to be healthy.[3] So it's not surprising that although we eat around 800 calories a day less than we did in the 1950s, we are still gaining weight. We've been distracted into thinking it's what we eat that makes the difference when it's really much more to do with what we do. Or don't do.

But before you start to panic, we're not talking about an obsessive gym habit, just a comfortable, unstressful exercise

3 European Food Information Council, 2000.

programme that fits in with the way you choose to live your life – yes, such a thing *does* exist!

Living by the rules

Another built-in failure factor a lot of diets have is that they tend to lay down an eating programme which is built around three meals a day. They can't be too flexible because splitting the calorie allowance between four, five or six meals a day would get too complicated. And most diets are already complicated enough, so snacking is labelled a sin.

The most important factor in deciding when to eat is *hunger*, but that doesn't seem to come into this equation. Your body doesn't necessarily need to eat the number of meals the diet dictates and eating smaller amounts of food more regularly is probably a better way of keeping your metabolism up to speed (like stoking the fire frequently rather than ignoring it and then putting loads of logs on all at once). Once again, the laboratory rats seem to prove the point – apparently they stay slimmer if they are fed a set amount of food in six separate sessions a day rather than having it all in one go.

The diet food dilemma

Another problem human beings share is that we all have a tendency to fall for the 'see-food' diet. Our primitive genetic coding sometimes tells us to eat when food's available, just in case there's a shortage tomorrow – and if crispy, golden, succulent goodies confront us at every street corner, we don't always stop to ask our stomach if we are genuinely hungry.

Of course, this weakness has been fully exploited by the big diet companies and the supermarkets too. The shops are full of products claiming to be low-fat or low-calorie, but they aren't really the slimming solutions that they appear to be.

How would you define slimming food? An orange? An avocado? A chicken salad? Or is it a pre-packaged ready meal with low-fat written all over it that looks very much like the high-fat, deep-fried product we'd actually prefer to eat? Are we really going to change our eating habits permanently by drinking three imitation chocolate milkshakes every day for a month? Or are our bodies going to be even more confused when we finally give up the pretend party food and start introducing weird stuff like fish and tomatoes and brown rice?

False promises and fake food

In January 2000 nutritionist Dr John Briffa reported that a loaf of well-known slimming bread has the same number of calories as ordinary white bread; the reason it's only 28 calories a slice is because the slices are smaller than the slices on a normal loaf. And he discovered that the same was true for quite a few other slimming products. In fact, the soup he checked out was actually higher in fat than the regular version – but the portion was half the size.

Another problem with special diet foods is that, in order to make them taste as good as real food, a lot of sugar or chemicals have to be added. So a *low-fat* label often means *high sugar*. A *Sunday Times* article in February 1999 by Steve Farrar and Tom Robbins revealed that many leading slimming products (including diet drinks) are simply loaded with sugar which can be addictive as well as harmful; according to that same article, refined sugar consumption could be responsible for the deaths of 3000 British women a year from heart disease.

And as for the chemicals, well, that's a controversial subject and the jury is still out on a lot of them. But in the meantime it's safer to stick with the simplest and most natural basic ingredients instead of putting stuff into our bodies that we haven't learned to deal with.

So, weighing up the evidence, it seems that the best thing about diet meals is that they are much more expensive than real food so you probably can't afford to buy as many of them.

SO WHY DO WE KEEP DOING IT?

The great thing about banging your head on a brick wall is that it's so wonderful when you stop. Of course, you may already have caused yourself a permanent injury . . .

People with problems are anxious and afraid that things will get worse – so the one thing they are reluctant to do is change, which, of course, is exactly what they most need to do.

In spite of the fact that dieting makes them miserable and doesn't provide a permanent solution, it's familiar territory. It can also be expensive and difficult, and that gives them confidence. Desperate people will believe anything – and if nothing's worked in the past it's reasonable to assume that they have to try harder and spend more money next time around. Of course, this opens the door to a lot of bizarre and even fake diet plans, as well as the usual calorie cutters.

A non-existent slimming plan called the Deakin Diet recently netted more than £16,000 in its very first week of advertising. It promised dramatic weight loss through using miracle slimming granules which never materialised and the Australian businessman behind the scheme was sent to gaol. Now, that's extreme, but a recent National Food Alliance survey found 88 per cent of slimming advertisements were misleading and didn't comply with advertising industry codes.

There are plenty of amateurs in the market too, but the fact that some of the diet plans doing the rounds are non-profit-making doesn't make them any more effective. My favourite so far is the ice-cream diet. But although the idea that it could actually be a good idea to eat an ice-cream before each meal and two in the evenings is clearly the product of a lot of wishful thinking, I can see the sadness in it too.

If I could put across just one message to all these people I would tell them to learn to trust themselves again, rather than putting their faith in magic menus. Lighten Up teaches you that change can be an enjoyable process during which you are glad to take on fresh challenges and get a new perspective on your relationship to food and activity.

Fat cats

Nutritional science has pretty much concluded that dieting cannot possibly work. But news like that doesn't get as much airspace as the heavily hyped promotions for the latest and most popular diets. Slimmers have a tendency to blame themselves for everything, including the fact that they are stuck in a dieting trap that doesn't work, but the fact that dieting is such a hugely profitable business probably has more to do with it.

Like the Americans, we spend a fortune on desperately trying to lose weight. In 1991, 29 million serious dieters in the US lost 630 million pounds and gained 489 million pounds of it back. It's obvious that money can't buy results, yet dieting is the fifth-largest industry in America, currently worth around $33 billion and growing fast.

So it probably won't surprise you when I tell you that 95 per cent of people who go on a diet put the weight back on again when it's finished. The slimming business is founded on failure and if only 4–5 per cent of slimmers stay slim, that's great news for the industry. In fact, the best thing about diets from a commercial point of view is the fact that they don't work – so they can rely on repeat business.

Scoring a goal and losing the game

A lot of slimming companies justify their products by saying that they are simply meeting a need, but it's a need they helped to create. You start dieting to lose a little weight and the diet encourages you to think more about food and eating than you ever did before. It's so easy to become a serial dieter.

Most people don't do it once and then go off and get a life. No, they diet, regain the weight and go on another diet. Then they lose the weight again and put it on once more. Dieting is like scoring a goal but losing the game. You lose weight temporarily, but you've got so used to counting calories, weighing yourself and fantasising about forbidden foods that it's very hard to go back to the natural way of eating when you're hungry.

Dieting promotes obsessive behaviour and, if that's been your way of life for a long time, it may not be easy for you to give it up and do things differently. But fortunately, if you decide to stick with the serial dieting, you needn't worry about running out of diets. There are over 330,000 to choose from and new ones are invented every week.

Failure

A lot of people talk about dieting in terms of failure. And they always blame themselves, not the diet. But it's the dieting industry which has failed its customers. *The diet business works because the product doesn't.*

Diets encourage us to take on new habits (and they're not necessarily good ones), but most people return to familiar ways when the diet's finished. It's no good relying on a diet to change your life. You can only do that by changing yourself.

> I started dieting in my late teens although looking at photos of me then, I wasn't fat – in fact, I was playing National Basketball, so I was physically very fit. However, for the next decade I tried every new diet that came on the market. Occasionally I would lose weight, only to regain it and more. Valiantly I continued doing what I had always done and getting what I had always got: failure, low self-confidence and even lower self-esteem.
>
> Finally in my thirties, the light went on and I realised that if I wanted a different result I needed to do something different. I eventually discovered Lighten Up – it's an inspiring programme – and now that I've done it I use the word 'impossible' with great caution.
>
> Lindsey Sills

MAKING UP YOUR OWN MIND

How many people do you know who have lost weight and kept it off? For a few months after the diet finished? For more than a year? For the rest of their lives? You can probably count them on one finger. Like casinos, the slimming industry celebrates with the winners but quietly makes its profit from the losers.

But if you're ready for an alternative, you already have one. You were born with a natural, built-in weight control mechanism. Lighten Up simply helps you get back into the habit of listening to your amazing body again and getting to know when you're hungry, what to eat and when to stop.

THE CHALLENGE

If you've been counting calories or weighing portions of food, stop doing it – just for this week.

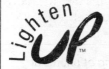 *Dieting won't keep you slim – it's what you do that makes the difference. Comfortable, regular exercise builds the muscle that burns the fat.*

CHAPTER THREE

THE DANGERS OF DIETING

What has dieting ever done for you?

If it had made you slim, fit and happy, we don't suppose you would be reading this. But maybe it's done more for you than you think.

Dieting's helped you to achieve a result. It may not be the result you wanted, but it's a result nevertheless. Maybe it's strengthened your self-image: you hoped to be slimmer, but now you know you're probably an overweight person through and through. Maybe you had some doubts about your identity, but now you know you're a weak-willed person with a food addiction. Maybe you needed to read your horoscope every morning to see how you were going to cope with the day, but now you just look at the scales instead and take it from there. And maybe your maths has improved because every time you forget your calculator you have to do some complicated arithmetic before you know what you're allowed to eat.

But, best of all, it's brought you to this point where you've said to yourself: 'I'm ready to do something different.'

IN THE SHORT TERM . . .

What are you missing?

Diets teach slimmers to look at food as dangerous calorie clusters rather than sources of energy and health. According to the diet books, a nourishing bowl of cereal is just thinly disguised cellulite. Because we get so concerned about what we shouldn't eat instead of what our bodies need, it's easy to lose sight of what we might be missing out on.

I already mentioned the B vitamins and magnesium that may be lacking if we start severely restricting what we eat but there are lots of other essential vitamins and minerals we need to keep us sane and active. A study at Rutgers University[1] analysed some of the most popular diet books and found that a number of them, including the Atkins, F Plan, Scarsdale, Carbohydrate Cravers, Pritikin and Stillman diets, were seriously deficient in vitamins, minerals or fibre.

Confusion rules

If somebody actually set out to invent a range of foods designed to contradict everything we know about good nutrition and disrupt the metabolism at the same time they could probably market it as a complete diet system. The main criteria seem to be:

★ Plenty of sugar to compensate for any fat reduction, provide empty calories and promote sugar addiction.
★ Artificial additives to make the food look and taste edible and confuse the body.
★ Meal substitutes that are just like sinful snacks (chocolate biscuits and milkshakes, for example) so they reinforce unhealthy eating habits and make sure we don't get out of the habit of grabbing a Mars bar instead of lunch.

---

1 Dr Paul La Chance and Michelle Fisher, Department of Food Science at Rutgers University.

A diet to die for

We originally wanted to call this book *A Diet to Die for*. 'That's too depressing,' the publishers told us.

'But dieting *is* depressing,' we said.

'Lighten Up isn't about dieting, it's about being in control of your weight,' they reminded us. We realised they had a point and changed the title.

That book title first came to mind when we were thinking of the really desperate victims of dieting, the growing number of people with eating disorders. The British Eating Disorder Association estimates that at least 90,000 people were treated for anorexia or bulimia in 2000 and this is thought to be just the tip of a very large iceberg. Many cases are ignored and untreated, particularly among young men, in spite of the fact that these are serious conditions. Anorexia has one of the highest mortality rates of any psychiatric illness.

I'm not saying that all eating disorders are caused by dieting, it's not as simple as that, but bulimics and anorexics are the extreme end of the spectrum that starts with calorie counting and worrying about your weight. Eating disorders are frightening and dangerous for the victims as well as for their families. It's a terrible thing to see someone you love disappearing – sometimes literally. Anorexia and bulimia are not normal behaviour, but neither is dieting. They are all forms of obsession, it's just that some forms are more extreme than others. Which is why I worry when we hear about ten-year-olds counting calories instead of being encouraged to walk to school or join a dancing class.

Dieting teaches you to spend your life thinking about food. It's a waste of mental energy and denies you one of the great pleasures of life, which is eating. Whether a diet tells you to cut out the steak or the chips, the one thing they all have in common is that they get you into the habit of thinking about food even when you aren't hungry.

Feeding the obsession

If one diet isn't working for them, people are often already on the lookout for the next one. They are so used to thinking constantly about what they want to eat and what they can't eat that it becomes an obsession. And you know what happens with obsessions – they feed on themselves and grow. And the bigger the obsession, the harder it is to break.

Diets just make you more and more aware of what you're eating – you start to think of food as 'good' and 'bad', you obsess about what you are and aren't 'allowed' to eat – and a very common result is that diets actually make people *put on* weight. Think about it – we bet it's happened to you at least once.

Memory loss

A study by the Institute of Food Research in 1999 showed a link between dieting and brainpower. It was already well known that dieting can make people depressed, and that's hardly surprising when you consider that it's all about low self-esteem and poor self-image. But the latest study discovered that women on crash diets suffer from memory loss and slow reactions. Apparently the mental malfunctioning was due to the brain's preoccupation with hunger, body shape and other diet-related thoughts.

So that explains it. These people go on a diet to lose weight and instead of making them thinner it simply impairs their memory so the next time they want to lose weight they've already forgotten that dieting doesn't work and they go on a diet . . .

I started dieting in my late teens with a diet of 1000 calories per day. I let myself eat what I wanted – as long as it was within the 1000 calorie limit. I weighed everything meticulously, taking my notebook and calorie counter everywhere with me. I lost weight. Over and over again. But I never quite reached my target before breaking the diet and gradually regaining the weight. I went through several cycles like this gaining and losing weight, always returning to the same 1000 calorie diet and always falling back to my pre-diet weight – plus just a little more.

My last diet was a fat-free one. I was training incredibly hard and eating very little or no fat. I certainly lost weight and I got the lean look I was after. But I was completely obsessed with food and

continued

my periods had stopped. I couldn't keep going and around Christmas time I started eating again. But it wasn't normal eating, I was bingeing hard. I planned to go back on the diet after Christmas but I couldn't do it. The thought of a chocolate biscuit would come into my head and I would buy a packet and eat the whole lot in one sitting. I felt terrible. I wasn't sure what was controlling me – my head, my body, or food. It was a compulsion I couldn't escape. I was frightened of being hungry.

I knew one thing for sure: I was never ever going to diet again. And that was the point when I realised that if I hadn't started dieting in the first place I might well have stayed at the weight I started at. I was angry at myself for being so obsessed with food. I would read back over my diaries and feel bad about giving myself such a hard time, and then give myself a hard time for giving myself a hard time.

Eventually, having been from one extreme to the other, I knew deep down that I needed to start being kinder to myself. My focus on food had led me to become so obsessed with it that all I did was eat. I know now I needed to focus on trying to get happy and put food in its place.

When I came across the Lighten Up programme it made absolute sense to me. I realised that I had found some techniques which would put food in its place, and put me back in touch with how food made me feel. I was thrilled to find that I got happier and even slimmer. My mistake in the past was believing that losing weight would make me happy. Whereas simply by becoming a happier person, I became slimmer.

Loraine Ilott

LONG TERM DAMAGE

Set-point theory

There's an interesting theory about how our bodies really control our weight, and it categorically disproves the 'calories in equals calories out' proposition that those doctors at Michigan University came up with in the 1930s. The 'set-point' theory seems to show that the body is actually capable of regulating weight to within a very narrow margin, almost regardless of how many calories we've actually ingested.

Scientists believe that the body has a set point around which it balances weight against calorie intake with amazing precision. When animals and human beings are force-fed, or starved for a while, they always revert to their original weight when they go back to eating normally. But in spite of the fact that the body can regulate weight so precisely, people still get fat because they can change their set point.

It seems that it takes a long time to change your set point. After six months on a high-fat diet rats don't go back to their original weight when they are given low-fat food again. They settle down at a much higher weight, so it looks as though their set point has changed. But if they live on a high-fat diet for *less* than six months they return to their previous lower weight.

Fat genes

Research is still being done on this but it seems quite likely that different people have different set points, which is bad news for people whose set points are tuned too high. The famous studies[2] of the Pima Indians in Mexico show that even if you do have a high set point, you can still stay slim by taking plenty of exercise and eating healthy food. The Pimas, a hard-working farming community, were generally slim and healthy until their lifestyle changed and they moved to a more sedentary life on a reservation with fast-food outlets. This unlucky tribe now has a much higher obesity rate than the rest of the North American population whose lifestyle they share – so it looks as though they have a genetic tendency towards a higher set point.

But another branch of the Pimas, down in Mexico, have stuck with their traditional low-fat, high-vegetable diet, which they work hard to produce, and they are still fit and wiry.

The lesson we learn from the Pima Indians is that, regardless of your set point, the key to staying slim is a natural, un-processed, low-fat diet with plenty of exercise.

2 Dr Claude Bouchard, Laval University, Quebec, Canada.

But why should some tribes and some individuals have a higher set point than others? It seems that they have more fat cells and larger ones, too. Fat cells are like balloons: they can inflate and deflate. We get fatter by filling the ones we have and then adding new ones – and once you've added them, you can't get rid of them, you can only inflate or deflate them.

There can be huge differences between the numbers of fat cells people have. A slightly obese person has 25–30 billion fat cells, a moderately obese person has 60–100 billion and a massively obese person can have 300 billion or more. Obviously, the more fat cells you have, the easier it is to fill them, but if you've ever been seriously overweight and you suspect you have billions of fat cells – *it doesn't matter.* Whether you were born with more fat cells than other people, or whether you created them yourself by overeating – *it doesn't matter.*

What matters is that with healthy diet and exercise you can deflate those fat cells so you'll never know you've got them.

Some of us, like the Pima Indians, were designed to live in tougher times, but no matter what your personal blueprint may be, a healthy diet and regular activity is all it takes to be slim and healthy. Permanent dieters, exercise addicts and people with anorexia and bulimia spend hours of effort every day trying arbitrarily to rewire their personal circuits. But they're battling against themselves and they're not going to win.

DON'T DIET

There's still a lot we don't know about our set points and fat cells. But everything we've learned so far makes it clear that commercial diets are bound to interfere with our delicate natural balance –

★ By shocking our bodies into burning muscle instead of fat and damaging our ability to burn calories.
★ By stimulating our bodies into filling up our fat cells every time we come off a diet.

continued

- ★ By putting us at risk of not getting the vitamins and minerals we need to turn carbohydrates into energy rather than fat.
- ★ By encouraging us to rely on dieting rather than exercising and building up more calorie-burning lean tissue.
- ★ By restricting the range of food we might naturally eat when a varied diet is our best way of getting all the vitamins, minerals and fibre we need.
- ★ By selling us 'diet' foods which are often high in additives and sugar, and low in essential nutrients.

WHAT'S THE ALTERNATIVE?

I think we must have made our point by now that Lighten Up is not about dieting. We have a strong feeling that if something's going to work, it's got to be positive. Once you start avoiding things (especially when they're an essential part of life, like food) there's only one way to go and that's down. If you're an alcoholic you can join AA and live a perfectly happy life without it. You can get by without cocaine or heroin or tobacco. But every day you have to face the fact that you've got to eat to stay alive. And if every meal is a stressful experience for you right now, are you prepared to put up with that for the rest of your life?

THE CHALLENGE

Instead of asking, what am I doing to myself, open your diary and write down this question: 'What *could* I do *for* myself?' Refer back to it every day for the next few days and, if any answers come to you, write them down as well.

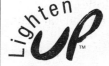

You are a unique and complex human being but a diet is a rigid, simplistic set of rules which will probably make your weight more unstable.

CHAPTER FOUR

SLIMMING FROM THE HEAD DOWN – HOW LIGHTEN UP WORKS

What stops you from being as slim as you'd like to be?

WHY LIGHTEN UP WORKS

Lighten Up works simply because human beings are so complicated. However overweight or overanxious about being overweight you are, you are more than a cluster of fat cells.

Wait and see what works for you

A friend of mine was an opera singer with a beautiful voice but less than beautiful teeth. When she landed her first big role, the producer gave her an ultimatum: get the teeth fixed or get back in the chorus. Phobic as she was about dentists, she signed up for the necessary orthodontics but during her final session something awful happened. The dentist was using a drill on one of the new crowns when, suddenly, something gave way in her inner ear.

She came to see me afterwards and she was desperate. She could still hear, but she couldn't judge pitch or tonality any more, even when she sang. Her 'ear' had quite literally gone. After a flood of tears she suddenly got up and marched out. I knew her well enough to know she was going to fix the problem; her mind was set on her opening night, still three weeks away and she was determined to be note-perfect. I didn't think about it again until we got complimentary tickets in the post. I hadn't heard from her in the meantime, so when the curtain went up *I* was nervous but she sounded perfect. Afterwards I asked her how she fixed it.

'I went for the scattergun approach,' she said. 'I saw a psychiatrist, a faith healer, a neurosurgeon and I had some acupuncture. Oh, and my GP gave me some antibiotics in case it was an infection.'

'So what worked?'

'I don't know. My body's never let me down before so I just gave myself a range of options and let nature take its course. I knew I would be all right on the night.'

Does that sound random? Not really. If you make sure you have all the information you need and take all the right steps to solve a problem, you can sit back and trust your body and mind to make the necessary adjustments. Which is exactly how this book works. We give you the information and we show you how to make the changes. Some of the Lighten Up techniques will work better for you than others. You won't know which ones will make you slimmer until you've tried them. All you have to do is follow the eight week course and expect to see the difference.

Energy, Eating and Exercise

The failure of diets shows us that concentrating on just one aspect of slimming – such as what you eat – is never going to work. Dieting alone is as likely to be as successful as do-it-yourself liposuction – though perhaps *slightly* less dangerous. It's safer and more effective to go for a holistic approach and tackle weight loss from all three important angles: Energy, Eating and Exercise. If you're going to succeed, you need to be totally prepared.

And energy, or the motivation that you put into changing shape, is the most important part of the equation. Nobody else can do it for you. If you want to reach your true, slim, fit, healthy, glamorous potential, you are going to have to learn to trust yourself. Of course you'll want to make some changes to your eating and exercise patterns but to start with it's your brain you'll be exercising. The key to success is getting your head around the changes you want your body to make.

Slimming from the head down

Lighten Up is often called 'slimming from the head down'. And as you start to loosen up your thinking, you will find your body becoming more flexible as well. Lighten up your mind and the weight will start to shift.

Permission to lose weight

It's no good expecting your body to change unless you first get permission from your brain. In fact, you need more than permission, you need co-operation as well. Your weight is a delicate balancing act and unless you get that balance right, your chances of success are slimmer than you'll ever be.

Self-control

Admit it, those were the words you didn't want to hear. But what I mean by self-control isn't the constant battle against yourself that you are probably very familiar with. By self-control I mean being in control of your own situation so that you're free to put your energy into generating the changes your body wants you to make.

Time to change

Change can be scary, but it's not usually as difficult as most people think it will be. Because we often have quite a bit of resistance to the idea of change, we deliberately frighten ourselves about it so we have an excuse to maintain the status quo. Which, of course, is another reason why diets don't work. It's not just your body that tries to hang on to the shape you've been for the past year or so, your brain is pretty conservative too. Some over-weight people have their personality and their relationships with other people all tangled up with their size and self-image. If their body shape changes, so does the shape of everything else and then life starts to get complicated. They might have to start having sex again, or running in the parents' race at the school sports day or even start living life instead of watching it go by. And that sort of thing takes a lot of effort.

I know so many people who are secretly determined not to change. They pay lip service to the idea, but they aren't keen on even going through the motions – especially when the motions take the form of exercise. Of course, dieting is perfect for you if that's how you feel because you don't actually have to do any-thing at all. *Dieting is about not doing rather than doing.*

In fact, the easiest thing you can do with this book is noth-ing. When you get to the eight-week course you could look at the exercises and tell yourself you'll try them later. Or you could compromise and do them half-heartedly. But you'll only really do them if you start doing them straight away. And you might just as well, because actually, it's no big deal. All the changes in this book are ones your body's been dying to make anyway.

The slimming instinct

Once out of the dieting trap, you're free to run your own life and make your own decisions about the shape you're in. You'll be working with your body rather than against it and this is where intuition comes in.

I'm not particularly New Age, but I do know that intuition is probably the single most important slimming tool. It's not mystical, or even mysterious, it's about making more use of the super-sophisticated piece of software that we have built into us. We don't use our brains positively enough when we waste our mental energy on things that are going wrong. And we insult our own intelligence with lists of arbitrary rules, which often contradict a lot of what we know, deep down, about the way our body works.

Set-point theory makes it clear that everybody's body and everybody's metabolism is different – but that we have the power to change. Whether you are a Pima Indian or Olive Oyle, it's your birthright to be *slim, fit and healthy*. But if you want to be the size and shape you were meant to be, you have to start from where you are. It means paying some attention to yourself and listening to your stomach, and if you're prepared to do that (it's going to take time and patience) you can be your own best friend and adviser.

The trouble is that it's easier to follow rules than it is to trust yourself. We've been taught to follow rules ever since our first day at school (and probably long before that) and the advantage is that it means not having to take responsibility for things that don't work. As long as we stick to the rules, it's not our fault. But do you really want someone else telling you what to eat, and when, for the rest of your life? You can't solve an internal problem like your weight with an external solution like a diet that somebody else has drawn up for you.

A change of mind

For years it's been accepted that our brains deteriorate as we get older and that we lose our mental agility along with our brain cells. Scientists believed that no new cells could be added to the human brain during adulthood, no matter how much new learning or experience was being acquired. Of course that would be a great excuse for not bothering to make changes in our lives, but I never believed the theory was true. My work with athletes (of all ages) has shown me that the brain has almost no limits – and if the brain can change, the body will follow.

And now some very recent research[1] in California and Sweden has discovered large numbers of new cells developing in

1 *Brain Cell Regeneration*
    (i) 'Research Turns Another "Fact" Into Myth', A. J. S. Rayl, *The Scientist* 13 [4]: 16, February 1999.
   (ii) Notebook, 'Challenging Fate', *The Scientist* 12 [22]: 35, November 1998.
  (iii) P. S. Erikson et al, 'Neurogenesis in the adult human hippocampus', *Nature Medicine*, 4: 1313–7, November 1998.

people's brains, in the area involved with learning and memory. The latest data also suggests that learning new things will stimulate the development of those new brain cells.

Of course, our brains prefer the status quo, just as our bodies do. But it's actually possible for the mind to make huge leaps and changes, and science now seems to be proving that this is true. It looks as though we have much more control over our own brains than we thought – so there's absolutely no reason why we can't change our own thought patterns and behaviour patterns. We

---

For years I knew my eating obsessions were in my head. I was the prisoner of my bad eating habits, endless conflicting emotions and food obsessions. For years I'd been yo-yo dieting, going through thin times and fat times, and getting more and more depressed about it.

Then I started the Lighten Up programme and things began to change. Because Lighten Up tackled what was going on in my head and that's where I made the first changes. My weight started to come off slowly but surely. It was great not worrying about weighing myself like I used to. My clothes alone were a testament to how well I was doing. At work the compliments were flowing in and my family and friends couldn't believe the change in me.

I feel like shouting from the treetops, I have seen the light and want to tell all those sad, unhappy people that there is an answer. Losing weight doesn't have to mean misery, deprivation, counting points or calories, red or green days or even sweating buckets in the gym. Just normal healthy eating patterns.

I wake every day, happy with myself. No more blue days worrying about getting the zip done up on my uniform or how I'll look at the next family gathering. Now I'm just me, happy, confident, positive and enjoying life to the full. Lighten Up makes so much sense – it was all so obvious – and surely so much easier than conventional dieting. The ideas are all so simple, anyone can easily take them on board.

Angela Smith

---

aren't just stuck with what we've got and we don't need to be victims of the way we're made.

We can, literally, change our minds.

The construction kit

A lot of change programmes are sold as toolkits but we always think that sounds as though you are trying to fix something that's gone wrong. There's nothing wrong with you, your body and mind are working brilliantly in spite of the fact that you may not have been giving yourself as much support and respect as you deserve.

Lighten Up is more of a construction kit than a toolkit – it's for building extensions to your current operating system and giving yourself more living space.

We'll be giving you lots of up-to-date information about how your body and mind actually work and what you need to eat and do to keep yourself fit and healthy. We'll also be suggesting a lot of different ways to get back in tune with yourself and gain control over your weight. When you know all the facts and you're aware of all the options, you are in the strongest possible position to trust your gut feeling and do what you know is right for you.

Of course, in Part Two, when we go through the Lighten Up Eight-week Course, you'll be learning all sorts of useful stuff – like how to eat when you're hungry and how to know what you really need. But by the time we get to Week Eight, it will seem so normal that you'll be doing it without thinking about it – and that's when you'll have the time to start enjoying your meals again and feeling good about yourself.

Beware – or just be aware?

Now this is quite contrary to what most slimming programmes tell you. The standard advice is that you are your own worst enemy – at every turn you're likely to succumb to a doughnut or veer off to the pub and down eight pints before stopping for a curry on the way home. We don't think that's true and we think the reason we often let ourselves down is actually because we don't really trust ourselves at all. We assume that what we shouldn't do is what we really want to do. How many times have you eaten a chocolate or drunk a glass of wine knowing, even as you swallowed it, that you didn't really want it? But because you thought you weren't allowed to do it, something told you to assert your right to that piece of pleasure.

More science

Science is beginning to take seriously the possibility that some people instinctively know how much they need to eat and automatically stop when they've had enough. At Lighten Up we're always pleased to hear about these studies, although I already know from my work with slimmers and non-slimmers over the years that we all have this ability. It's just that some of us have tuned it out and started eating for lots of reasons other than hunger. Reasons that seemed good to us at the time, but which have resulted in us becoming overweight and unhappy in the long term.

In 1999, a nutritional scientist, Barbara Rolls at Pennsylvania State University in the US, found evidence that 'Some adults regulate food intake based on their bodies' physiological signals'. A group of male volunteers were given yoghurts with either added fat or added carbohydrate. The yoghurts looked and tasted the same and some of the men ate the same amounts of both the higher-calorie and the lower-calorie yoghurt. But some of them didn't. One group automatically, and without knowing why, ate less of the higher-calorie yoghurt. The volunteers with this instinct for which yoghurt was healthier were always normal-weight men with no hang-ups about their weight; they seemed to have a built-in, subconscious calorie counter. The men who couldn't distinguish between the fatty and less fatty yoghurts were either overweight or worried about their weight.

The men with the healthy attitude towards food and towards themselves apparently had an internal mechanism that could detect the energy content of food fast enough to allow them to adjust their intake.

The really great news I have found out and proved to be true over and over and over again is that we can *all* rediscover that innate ability to know how much to eat and when to stop.

The greatest diet in the world is to eat when you're hungry and finish before you feel too full. It's the natural intelligence that was built into us when we were born.

Believe it and achieve it

Lighten Up goes beyond positive thinking into positive action. And actions speak louder than words, which is why this book is full of things you can do to change your life, not later but *now*.

THE CHALLENGE

See how flexible you are. Think of a minor problem you have right now – it might be your weight, or it might be a deadline at work or an argument with a friend. Get your notebook and write down five things you could do to improve the situation. Then pick the one that scares you most and give it a go.

It doesn't matter whether it works or not. We just want you to see how it feels to change your mind – and your perception of yourself.

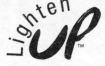 Lighten Up will give you the information you need to make your own slimming choices together with the techniques to make them happen. The rest is up to you.

CHAPTER FIVE

HABITS

How did you get into the habit of being overweight?

IF YOU DO WHAT YOU'VE ALWAYS DONE, YOU'LL GET WHAT YOU'VE ALWAYS GOT

Have you been dieting for ages? Or are you just living your life in the wrong body? However things are, you're probably used to them being that way. Maybe you sometimes get close to the weight you want to be, but do you ever really believe you can stay there?

If it's not your first time, I want to ask you to think carefully about what you really want and what you expect to get. This isn't about counting calories, or food combining, or eating before five o'clock. That's just rules and rules are a piece of cake. Which, as you've often been told, makes you fat.

Being overweight is one of the saddest of life's problems because it's the one you can't hide. If you're overweight you can't stop everybody looking at you and wondering why you're the way you are. 'Is he depressed? Is she lazy? Is he unmotivated? Doesn't she have a sex life? Doesn't he care? Isn't her health suffering? Is he just a slob?'

Everybody else can keep their difficulties under their hat, but you wear yours on your hips and thighs. Standing in the bus queue you can't tell a wife beater from a child abuser or even a potential mass murderer – or a schizophrenic from a burnt-out trader on cocaine. Yet the overweight businesswoman who has gained a few pounds through a few bad habits has her problem clearly on display.

Normal people with fat habits

Habits are like deep holes, easy to fall into and hard to get out of. But the great thing about them is that they are only bits of behaviour that you do. They aren't part of you, they aren't part of your personal blueprint and they have nothing to do with your real identity.

Years ago I had a client called Harry who had been overweight for twenty years, ever since his marriage broke up, in fact. 'Of course,' he said, 'you've only got to look at my family to see that the odds are stacked against me.' He pulled a picture out of his wallet: his nephew's graduation showed a collection of plump lookalikes, lined up and looking proud. But there was one older man who seemed to be in much better shape than the others.

I pointed to him. 'Who's that?'

'My father. He had a heart attack five years ago and since then he's been under doctor's orders to change his lifestyle. He's taken up walking and tennis, and he's started eating fruit for breakfast.' Harry's expression told me very clearly how abnormal he thought this particular behaviour pattern was.

He caught my eye. 'Don't start lecturing me about my lifestyle. Dad didn't have any choice; it was change or die. Anyway, he's retired so he's got more time than the rest of us for the healthy food and exercise routines.'

'Well,' I said, 'suppose you just swapped a few of your bad habits for some better ones? That way it needn't take up any extra time. You could cycle to work, for example, and perhaps do a few exercises while you watch *Match of the Day*?'

Harry went on our eight-week course and steadily lost weight. But it wasn't until I met him in the street a year later that he told me about his personal turning point. 'You know what clicked with me at that first meeting we had?' he said. 'I remember you saying I could swap some of my bad eating habits for some more positive ones. Well, the funny thing was that as soon as I started thinking about my lifestyle and my weight as bad habits, it didn't seem quite so difficult to do something about them. They weren't part of me any more, just some behaviour I could modify a bit.'

I learned a lot from that. If Harry could change, anybody can change – and the key seems to be realising that you aren't a fat person. You're just a normal person with some fat habits.

Beginning to break those habits

If you don't like exercise, if you eat popcorn instead of proper meals, if you give yourself a hard time most of the time, these are just things you've taught yourself to do with a bit of encouragement from your family and friends. You've trained yourself to be the person you are, you've practised for it and you've succeeded. But now it's time to put the same effort, energy and dedication into being something else.

It probably took you a long time to build up the complex pattern of habits that make up your life. In the case of the good ones (like cleaning your teeth) it's time well spent. But it actually takes more time and dedication to be consistently, destructively dysfunctional than it does to be a winner. After all, good habits are often self-reinforcing. You smile at someone and they smile back. But being a consistent grouch (for example) takes a bit more effort.

★ So the first step towards positive change is to recognise the effort you've put into that habit you wish you didn't have.
★ The second step is to recognise that you could redirect that effort into setting up some new and positive habits, which could change your life for the better *for ever*.

Take time to change

The third step is to accept that it took you a long time to be such an accomplished couch potato/negative thinker/junk food addict and give yourself the time you need to change.

If something you do has really got a hold on you (like being seriously inactive, for example) don't expect it to disappear overnight. Just start chipping away, habit by habit, and keep your eye on the goal of becoming slimmer, fitter and healthier.

Take a break without the KitKat

Of course you can't consciously change things you don't know about, so the first thing we'll be getting you to do in Part Two of this book is to keep a diary. But it's not a calorie-counting diary, it's a pattern-spotting diary. We want you to learn more about you and how you are going to change. Because then you can start living life differently.

Let's suppose that you have a habit of overeating when you are stressed. We know that's only one possibility and there are lots of others, but let's just use it as an example because stress eating is so normal as to be almost obligatory if you're overweight – though that doesn't make it a good idea! We want you to imagine what it would be like to *take a day off* from your habit. Imagine yourself having a really boring day, for example, but as the hours tick slowly by, instead of reaching for a snack, you get up and do some deep breathing, or go for a walk, or phone a friend, or stroke the cat. And if you're stuck at work, take a couple of minutes to imagine how much fun you're going to plan into your next free time.

Perhaps you can't imagine getting through a whole day like that, so make it a bit easier. How about just an afternoon, or an hour, or even five minutes? The point is, if you can do it for a few seconds, you can do it.

You can't take time off from being you, but you can take a break from doing all the things you wish you didn't do.

Remember the reason

Every habit starts for a reason. And the reason may be a good one at the time, but perhaps it doesn't make sense any more.

Babies only eat when they are hungry but most of us have gradually been persuaded to eat for other reasons. It's no wonder that food holds a vice-like grip on our emotions and that our relationship with it is complicated. And often the food we eat in non-hunger situations is sweet and fattening and leaves us feeling miserable and bloated. Whatever we eat when we aren't hungry gets turned into fat and stored for later.

You were probably trained to abuse your digestive system from an early age. Perhaps your mother was worried about you not eating, or your teacher tried to comfort you with a Smartie when you grazed your knee, or you were given chocolate as a reward for doing something well. None of those agendas is relevant to you now. Perhaps they never were. But are you still living them to the letter?

And it's not only personal problems that produce negative patterns. Although it ended half a century ago, a lot of our eating habits have been influenced by the war. Our parents or grandparents can remember rationing, even if we can't. Food was short, anything sweet was in great demand and for years afterwards children were taught to empty their plates if they wanted pudding. Of course, I'm not suggesting we blame our excessive weight on Hitler or anyone else, just pointing out that if we're still living by somebody else's rules it's time to ditch them and live by our own.

But the most difficult habits to break are those we've invented for ourselves and gradually become dependent on. We know very well that eating a HobNob – or even a packet of them – won't bring back a boyfriend or make our life more exciting, or even improve our job prospects. But a few biscuits and a cup of tea are very effective comforters in the short term. The trouble is that these little things easily become indispensable institutions.

There are so many things we do that we don't need to any more. We just haven't bothered to tell our brains there are better alternatives.

BRING ON THE SUBSTITUTES

One of the things I did with Harry right at the beginning was to get him to draw up a habit list. It was just a piece of paper, divided into two columns. It didn't take him long to fill up the right hand side, but the left looked pretty empty.

Good Habits	Bad Habits
Eating 3 pieces of fruit a day	Egg Mac Muffin for breakfast most days
Drinking lots of water	Eating crisps while I watch football
Getting plenty of sleep	Sugar in my tea (I drink a lot of tea)
	Going out for a curry whenever I have a couple of beers
	Always saying yes to second helpings of pudding
	Driving to work instead of walking
	Doing the crossword instead of getting away from my desk at lunchtime
	Lying in on Sundays instead of football practice

'OK,' I said. 'Now take another look at that column on the left and see if you can add to it at all.'

He laughed and shook his head so we picked up the paper and started writing in the Good Habits column:

> Cleaning teeth regularly
> Wearing clean clothes
> Walking the dog last thing at night
> Getting to work on time every day
> Being nice to the children

'Surely that doesn't count,' Harry said. 'Everybody does them and they've got nothing to do with losing weight.'

But, as I explained to him, they are still habits. Just because they are good habits we don't think about them, but they are the other side of the coin to all the negative habits we have. Harry's not unusual. If we thought about every single thing we did, life would be too complicated – if you actually stopped to consider how difficult it is to ride a bike you'd need training wheels again. Doing some things automatically is very useful and we depend on having a lot of good habits that keep us going from day to day, but there's no reason why we can't deliberately install a few new good habits and use them to help us control some of our negative ones.

Habit holes

Once you've climbed out of a habit hole, fill it up immediately. If you don't you're likely to fall right back in it again next time you trip over a problem, a piece of chocolate cake, or a bottle of wine. And the best way to fill a habit hole is with another habit – but this time, make it a positive one that helps you feel good and look good, too.

We were talking about habit holes on a Lighten Up course one evening and the group seemed to share a particular addiction: they all watched *EastEnders*. 'What's wrong with that?' I wondered.

'Well,' said one lady, 'I need something to do with my hands, because it's on as soon as I get in from work and I can't really relax. So I almost always have something to eat while it's on.'

And, of course, so did everybody else. In fact, the only difference seemed to be what they ate – it ranged from anything that was left over in the fridge (this counts as tidying up, apparently) to Mars bars and Marmite sandwiches. One of the men in the group had managed to crack this habit – but only by substituting a couple of beers for the taco chips he used to eat.

I challenged them to come up with a way of filling the *EastEnders* hole with something other than food and the next week they came back with a list of suggestions. Here are a few of the ones I can remember:

★ ironing
★ half an hour on the exercise bike, doing some stretches or lifting weights

- ★ having a manicure or a pedicure
- ★ having a facial or using pore-strips
- ★ moving the TV into the kitchen and preparing dinner at the same time
- ★ lying on the bed, totally relaxing
- ★ brushing the cat
- ★ giving your partner a back massage (you can watch it over his or her head)
- ★ slowly sipping water or herb tea

So, before you zap a habit you don't want, take a moment to make a list of good things you could put in its place. In fact, if you have a habit in mind at the moment, you might like to pause for a moment and make that list now.

It's a habit not a horoscope

When you re-label your overeating/under-exercising or negative thinking as just a bad habit, you take away its power to control your life. By truly understanding that it's not part of you, that it's just something you do, you put yourself in charge again. You can *choose* not to drink or smoke or procrastinate, even if you only make that choice for short periods to start with. And whenever you empty a bad-habit hole, even temporarily, you can fill it up with something positive instead.

Here's one we did earlier

I've had my own battle with habits that threatened to take over my life. For years I was a victim of my own obsession – I wanted to be perfect! I was a knowledge junkie and I read every book I could lay my hands on. But I also pushed my body too hard with over-exercising. I got to the point where there were not enough hours in the day to do all the reading and training I wanted to do. Eventually, of course, my body protested and my mind started to realise that my life was seriously unbalanced.

It started, like all bad habits, for a perfectly good reason. Having not achieved much at school, I was absolutely determined when I left that I was going to prove my teachers wrong and be the best I could be at everything. And that was OK – until it got out of control.

Once I realised what was happening (perhaps if I'd been keeping a diary or making lists I'd have noticed this pattern sooner) I was able to change. My mind was overloaded with information I didn't have time to use – and, as a result, I was missing the really urgent warning signals my body was trying to give me.

Listen to your body and exercise your mind

One of the most refreshing things I ever did was to stop taking in so much information and start using the knowledge that I actually had. Of course, I had already been using that knowledge from time to time, but not consistently. In particular, I remember realising, years ago, that losing weight means only eating when you are hungry. Then I had to tackle the problem of how to teach people to know the difference between hunger and boredom – or hunger and anxiety. Our bodies know what we need, but even those of us who really care about fitness and physical performance sometimes miss the messages our bodies send us.

I never used to get hangovers, but I do now (occasionally). A hangover is hard to ignore, but we often ignore the more subtle warning signs our bodies give us – pain when we over-exercise, discomfort when we overeat. If you really listen to your body, you'll discover that all the information you need is there – you just need to learn to trust it.

So don't take anything for granted. Just because you've been living this way for a long time doesn't mean it's right for you or that it's the only way to be. If it doesn't feel right, experiment with change.

Know what you know

And once you start to understand what a unique and valuable human being you are, you will soon be able to take the next step and start paying attention to all the valuable information, insights and instincts that are built into your amazing brain. You already have all the information you need to understand what is going on in your life and make the adjustments you want to make. But don't take our word for it – learn from our experience.

Good practice

Remember that the habit-changing part of the Lighten Up programme is like training to be a champion. If you're going to succeed in getting rid of the bad stuff in your life and refilling it with positive patterns, you need to keep at it. Making that list and appraising your life balance is the first good habit you should aim to install and then it's a question of practise, practise, practise.

When we learn a new skill the goal is to be able to do it without thinking about it and, of course, this is what many of you have achieved with your eating habits. No baby ever plopped out of the womb thinking, 'That was stressful, I need a Mars bar.' You weren't born reaching for Pringles as a reaction to stress, depression or boredom, so you just need to unlearn those habits.

THE CHALLENGE

Identify one of your eating habits and substitute it for something else. Choose something really minor – if you always have a raspberry yoghurt for lunch, pick a different flavour, or if you take two spoonfuls of sugar in your tea, make it one. See how the difference feels.

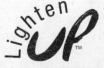

The Lighten Up programme helps you identify all the habits you have that affect your weight. You'll be getting rid of the ones you don't want and replacing them with new ones that will make the changes happen.

CHAPTER SIX

THE DIFFERENCE THAT MAKES THE DIFFERENCE

Do you think the way you look is really you?
Would you like to look different?

SEEING THE BENEFIT

Selling your dream

Lighten Up started about ten years ago when I first got curious about weight control and why it was such a problem. One of my first clients was a super-salesperson for a big computer company and I was always impressed when she had to fly off to Europe at short notice to address conferences of lesser salespersons. Even when it meant she had to miss her training sessions with me.

I was showing her a series of exercises to tone up her abdominal muscles one day when she suddenly said, 'You're breaking the golden rule, you know.'

My first instinct was to panic, but I didn't think I'd said or done anything politically incorrect. Then I noticed she was still smiling so I decided it couldn't be too serious. When I asked her what she meant, she said, 'Whenever you take me through these wonderful routines that are going to be so good for me, you always tell me how effective they are and how they've been tried and tested and all of that. But you never sell me the benefit!'

I was even more confused, so she explained. 'It's a classic sales technique. Never sell the customer the product. They already know what the product is. Sell them the benefit and then they can go on selling it to themselves. Otherwise, even if they buy it, they won't bother to use it. Now, if you were to tell me how good *I'm* going to look – or feel – rather than how great these exercises are you'd be much more likely to get my buy-in.'

Buying your dream

So no wonder my early attempts to sell exercise plans and diet sheets didn't get results – I was selling the product instead of the benefit. In fact, I was trying to impose a watered-down version of my own exercise and eating programme on other people – which is about as likely to be successful as trying to clone a sheep from an elephant. No matter how carefully I tailored things to each individual's lifestyle, age, weight, sex and level of fitness, I hadn't bothered to get them actually to buy into it.

PAIN AND PLEASURE

Although on reflection I've come to the conclusion that it's my job to teach *you* to sell *yourself* the benefits of slimming rather than trying to sell you the benefits myself – after all, you are the only person who really knows what it would mean to you to be slimmer, fitter and healthier for the rest of your life – that piece of sales advice taught me a lot. But deep down I still felt that the lucky people I was working with should be able to see for themselves the benefits of the exercise and eating plans I designed for them. After all, it wasn't as though there was anything wrong with the plans. They always worked for me.

Sitting in the café at the pool one day, I was reading through some exercise routines and thinking, 'If this were all I did in a day I'd be laughing – why the hell can't any of them stick with it?' Of course, what I hadn't taken into account was my personal weird factor.

Getting high on your own supply

I always loved exercise. In fact, when I was a child my parents and teachers used to wish I weren't quite so permanently active. Although I didn't know what it was, I realised from a very young age that there was a free endorphin rush to be had. I loved getting high on my own supply and I assumed that everybody else had made the same discovery.

One thing my parents and teachers did manage to drum into me – when they could keep me still for long enough – was the concept of value for money. Which was another reason why I could never understand why people would spend so much money on health club membership and diets that they would abandon after a few months, or weeks – or even faster than that.

So what was going on? I might have stayed in the dark for a long time if a friend of mine (it takes someone who knows you really well to tell you the important stuff) hadn't asked me a question. This was a guy I'd known since school – not one of my super-fit colleagues – and the question was this: 'Why do you think people don't take enough exercise?'

'I don't know,' I said irritably. I'd been asking myself the same question over and over without getting a sensible answer.

'Because they don't like it,' said Dave. 'I don't like it myself – you know that. Most of us aren't like you and that bunch of wannabe gladiators you work with. So if you truly mean to help people lose weight you'd better join the real world.'

I was shocked, but it was obviously true. In fact, I was so shocked that I started taking other people a lot more seriously than I ever took myself after that. I realised that I'd probably been treating my clients as animated bundles of muscles and fat cells that needed rebalancing, rather than as human beings with minds of their own. I simply hadn't understood that a lot of people didn't like exercise.

And that was when I fathomed that *people only become slimmer and stay slimmer when the slimming process itself gives them pleasure and being overweight gets too painful.*

Pleasure and pain

The problem is that for most people dieting is painful and so is exercise. For example, take a look at this list of words and underline the ones you associate with dieting and exercising to lose weight (and we mean *actually* underline them in this book – it's yours after all. Get a pen).

Achievement
Anorexia
Antisocial
Anxiety
Appetite
Ashamed
Attraction
Attractive
Beauty
Bed
Binge
Bonny
Bony
Boring
Boy
Bulge
Bulimia
Burden
Burn
Cakes
Calorie
Calorie Control
Celery
Cheating
Chocolate
Choice
Christmas
Clinic
Clothes
Club
Comfort

Confidence
Cottage cheese
Couch Potato
Counter
Counting
Cuddly
Dancing
Date
Denial
Depression
Deprivation
Deserving
Diet
Difficult
Dinner
Discipline
Doctors
Drinking
Drugs
Dynamic
Eating
Eating Disorder
Elegant
Embarrassment
Empty
Endorphins
Energy
Enjoy
Excess
Excitement
Exhaustion

Failure
Family
Fashion
Fast
Feeling Good
Film Star
Firm
Fit
Fitness
Fitting In
Flirting
Food
Free
Fridge Magnets
Friends
Fruit
Frump
Fry-up
Full
Fun
Girl
Glamour
Glow
Grapefruit
Grill
Guilt
Gymnasium
Happy
Hard
Healthy
Heavy

Hedonism	Party	Success
Hips	Pleasure	Suffering
Holiday	Plump	Summer
Hollow	Popularity	Sweat
Home	Poverty	Sweets
Hopeless	Pregnancy	Swimsuit
Hot	Promise	Tablets
Hypnotism	Psychiatry	Target
Ill	Psychology	Taste
Image	Regular Meals	Tea
Impossible	Salad	Temporary
Insecurity	Scales	Temptation
Lettuce	School	Temptress
Life	Secret	Thin
Light	Security	Tight-assed
Lonely	See-Saw	Tired
Love	Self-delusion	Tomorrow
Lunch	Self-esteem	Treadmill
Lycra	Sensuality	Trial
Lying	Sex	Unfit
Magazines	Sex Appeal	Vegetables
Martyr	Shape	Vitality
Mature	Shopping	Vitamins
Measuring	Size	Voluptuous
Men	Skeletal	Waist
Milkshake	Skin Problems	Waste
Mirror	Skinny	Wealth
Misery	Sleep	Weekend
Model	Slim	Weighing
Monstrous	Slow	Weight
Mother	Sluggish	Winter
Motivation	Smell	Women
Muscles	Smoking	Work
New Year	Snack	Worry
Nutrition	Social	Wrinkles
Obsession	Stable	Young
Old	Starving	
Pain	Substitute	

If that little exercise shows that you associate quite a bit of pain with the process of slimming, you're probably not very surprised. No wonder your body's been protesting, it's probably hungry and stressed.

So don't despair. Slimming doesn't have to bring pain, deprivation and a downturn in your social life. You've just been doing the wrong sort of exercise, eating the wrong food and focusing on too much pain. It's not surprising you didn't stick with it for long. You'd have to be crazy to succeed.

In fact, we're amazed that people manage to stick with complicated, antisocial, fun-free diets for as long as they do. Not only are they depriving themselves of pleasure, they are often hungry as well – and that's uncomfortable in itself.

And you can diet for ever, if you have a will of steel and low social expectations, but you can't get away from the sheer deliciousness of chocolate mousse, strawberry shortcake and sticky toffee pudding. Every now and again, or even more often than that, a treacle tart is going to creep up on you. And there's nothing wrong with treacle tart once in a while. The fat problem happens when all you can think about is treacle tart and you don't get any joy out of a banana – or a cucumber sandwich.

The Lighten Up mission, if you choose to accept it, is to move away from the traditional pain and deprivation model of dieting. And you start immediately.

Feeling better instead of feeling good?

So you associate diet and exercise with pain, that's pretty clear, but being – or feeling – overweight causes pain as well. It makes you unhappy. Then, in a long-established pattern, you eat to comfort yourself. You're not sorting out the problem and learning to feel good, you're just making yourself feel very temporarily better. And the thing is, we've all got so deeply into the habit of anaesthetising ourselves against the minor aches and pains of life that we forget the alternative of feeling good for more of the time. Of course you can be high as a kite in a few seconds if you take the right drugs and you can lose ten pounds in a week if you go for the wrong diet, but the long-term effects of those actions on your body and your mind will be damaging. It's short-term thinking.

Reacting against the chemicals

We live in a fast-fix society and there are plenty of legal and illegal drugs around that will artificially adjust your chemical balance. If you're feeling low, anything from chocolate and alcohol to 'smart' drugs on prescription or class A drugs on the street will do the trick. But that's the point I'm making. It is a trick. You are just fooling yourself into thinking you feel better in the   short term.

Then, inevitably, that feeling will wear off and you'll need more of what will eventually make you feel bad. Because, unfortunately, the amount of relief we get from chemical quick fixes tends to be in proportion to the negative after-effects. As a general rule, the bigger the buzz, the deeper the downside.

We go out every day looking for pleasure and everybody can afford to buy it in small doses – a bar of chocolate, a beer, a cigarette or a prescription. And if you have enough money and disregard for your health, you can buy faster fixes from less obvious sources. But even the little legal remedies for unhappiness cause long-term damage and I promise you – you don't need them.

No wonder the demand for Prozac and just about every other designer drug is rising fast and there's an epidemic of illegal mind-altering substances available on the streets. Could there be a connection here with so many people being overweight and out of condition? After all, a lot of people who draw the line at drugs are quite happy to use food to make them feel better when they get bored, depressed, angry, irritated or stressed.

Remember that your brain is just trying to help you. When you feel bad, your brain doesn't like it and it comes up with suggestions to help you change the way you feel. And food (unless you have an even more compelling addiction like class A drugs or smoking) is usually the fastest option. Did you know that in the last five years 'comfort food' has become an officially recognised piece of terminology, a part of our language?

If food has ever made you feel better or distracted you from a problem, your brain will helpfully suggest that solution again – even if you're feeling bad because you ate too much. Your brain isn't concerned about the long term, it just wants to make you feel better right away.

So wanting to feel good and avoid pain are pretty obvious. And going for short-term fixes that make us feel better for a short while and worse in the long term is understandable too. But I often wonder why human beings are so brilliant at feeling bad that they get into that mess in the first place? Why can't we just be nice to ourselves and look after our bodies and respect our thoughts? Why do so many people put others first and neglect their own needs? I know a lot of sensible people who treat their cars and their pets better than they treat themselves. The cars get the right petrol and regular servicing, and the dogs get vitamins and petting and regular walks. The owner, meanwhile, eats junk food and neglects his bodywork.

The mother of all Catch 22s

So this is where it gets interesting. It seems that the main reason a lot of people feel bad about themselves and resort to comfort eating and inactivity is their low self-image. They don't feel good about themselves. But what happens when you have a low self-image *and* you take drugs or eat to make yourself feel better? When your temporary remedy wears off you not only feel worse, you also look worse. And so it loops round again.

We'll be showing you how to change all that.

SELF-IMAGE

How many people do you know who genuinely feel good about themselves? We don't know that many. That's why Lighten Up tackles the cause of the problem (your self-image) rather than the effect (how other people see you).

Things I hate about me

The first item on the low-self-image list is usually your appearance. I'm amazed by the number of people who don't like what they see in the mirror. I don't think I've ever met a man or a woman who didn't have at least two things they hated about the way they look, so apparently beauty isn't only skin deep after all.

We judge people, including ourselves, by appearances. We're bombarded with impossible images of anorexic, silicone-enhanced, Barbie-doll perfection when the average woman would seriously have to undereat, have a couple of ribs removed to reduce her waist and then replace her starved-away breasts with silicone to get anywhere near Barbie's statistics.

Pressure to be perfect

Everybody's worried. We are constantly reminded that being beautiful is more important than anything else in the world. We are told that in order to be happy, successful, respected and to have good relationships, we have to look good. And, sadly, the desire to be beautiful undermines our self-esteem because it values us by standards we can't control. Age catches up with everybody in the end – although if you're wealthy you can hold it at bay for a bit longer than everybody else.

Here are some alarming facts:

★ Over a twenty-year period, the *Playboy* centrefold lost 25 pounds until she weighed 18 per cent less than the medical ideal for her age and height. The weight of the fashion models plummeted even further to 23 per cent below that of ordinary women. In the Miss World contest a few years ago, the average contestant was *below* the US standard weight for anorexia according to height.

★ Recent BMA research found that many currently popular models and actresses only have 10–15 per cent of their body composition as fat compared with 22–26 per cent for a normal, healthy woman.

★ It's estimated that 85 per cent of Americans have dieted. Hundreds of thousands of other women are undergoing cosmetic surgery, stomach stapling and liposuction.

★ In the 1994 Galmour survey of 33,000 women, three-quarters of the respondents regardless of age, income and education, reported feeling overweight, although only one quarter could be classified as truly overweight.

★ In a study done in a hall of distorting mirrors it was found that women were much more likely to believe the mirror that made them look fatter than the mirror which accurately reflected their size or made them thinner.

And the tragic part of it is that as ideal women get smaller, real women get bigger, so the dissatisfaction gap is widening all the time.

People you don't know can ruin your evening

I remember when I first realised that superficial appearances could have profound effects. I was sitting in a bar, chatting to a girlfriend, when I noticed her attention wander. She was looking over my shoulder at a couple who had just walked through the door. They were a handsome pair, he was tall and tanned, and she was a willowy blonde. Then I noticed that she was wearing a very similar dress to the one my girlfriend had on. I turned to the girl I was with. 'He's good looking, isn't he?' I said magnanimously, assuming she'd be giving him the once-over.

She looked depressed. 'I didn't notice,' she said. 'That woman is wearing my dress and she looks better in it than I do.'

The evening didn't go well after that. Nothing I could say or do would make her happy again. 'How can you let somebody you don't even know make you miserable?' I asked her. 'That girl might be the most miserable cow in the universe. She might be broke, she might be out of work, she might be losing the love of her life. You don't know what she's really like, so why are you letting her get you down?'

LOOKING GOOD AND FEELING GOOD

So just suppose you could start to enjoy yourself more. And just suppose that by feeling better, you could start looking better too. We're not talking about turning into Pamela Anderson or Arnold Schwarzenegger, just becoming slim, fit and glowing with health. Would that do?

Well, here's how: get some regular, comfortable exercise into your daily routine and start enjoying your food again. And if you need some help with that, keep reading.

THE CHALLENGE

In your diary, draw up two columns. In one write down everything you don't like about taking exercise and healthy eating. In the other, write down the pleasure you would get from being slim and the pain you would feel if you stayed the way you are.

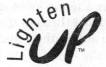

We are being sold some impossible images of physical perfection together with some equally impossible (or unpleasant and expensive) ways to achieve those ideals.

The way forward is actually very simple – if you want to be slimmer, fitter and healthier, you need to get more pleasure from eating healthy food and spend more time on physical activities that you really enjoy.

CHAPTER SEVEN

HOW TO GET WHAT YOU WANT

Why is it that some people succeed and others don't?

Working with both athletes and slimmers has shown us a lot of similarities between the winners in both worlds. Do you think you've failed as a slimmer? What about the rest of your life? Can you identify areas where you've made it and areas where you haven't?

Winners and losers

The reason why some people succeed and others don't is less to do with luck or talent than with how they think. Obviously, in sport, some people have more potential than others, but at the top, the physical gap between the champions and the also-rans is very small. It's the mindset that makes the difference.

Lighten Up started to happen when we discovered that small changes in the way we think can trigger big behaviour changes.

SUCCESS STRATEGIES

So what's the difference that makes the difference between success and failure? Well, there isn't *one*, there are quite a few.

Successful slimmers know when they've had enough

A lot of successful slimmers finally win their battle when they eventually get fed up with feeling fat and guilty. They've had enough so they are left with no choice but to change.

Successful slimmers are willing to take responsibility for what they eat and how they live. They don't need external rules; they eat and exercise according to how they feel. And they can do that because they are back in touch with what their bodies need.

Successful slimmers learn by their mistakes

Most things worth doing don't work brilliantly the first time. Whether it's riding a bike, driving a car, or having sex. So next time you don't get up in time to exercise, or you eat a few doughnuts too many, don't lose the plot. Learn something useful from it. Your lapses may be telling you something about what your body (or your mind) really needs. Lots of good things were discovered by accident – penicillin by Fleming, radium by Marie Curie, America by Columbus . . .

And, even if you *don't* get a mind-shattering revelation every time you pig out or slob out, instead of getting up and working out, just say to yourself: 'At least I'm going in the right direction – I still have choices.' After all, *what* you do is less important than your *response* to what you do.

It often happens that when everything's going well and you feel as though at last you're in control, getting fitter and firmer, an out-of-the-blue thunderbolt knocks you off course. You get flu, you pull a muscle and you can't exercise for a while. Your relationship ends, you lose your job and you get drunk or eat a box of popcorn and a curry. These things happen, they're an inevitable part of life, so don't overreact. If you get stressed and you overeat, or you're tired or bored and you overeat, just say, 'OK, that's what I did this time – what will I do differently next time?'

You can't control all the events and people in your life. You can't even control yourself all of the time. So when things go off track, as they will, accept it and look for a different way of dealing with the problem when it happens again.

Successful slimmers learn from their own achievements

I've studied a lot of successful people from all walks of life and you can do the same. Look for role models. When you're eating with thin people notice how fast (or more likely how slowly) they eat; when you live with thin people, check what they do that you don't. But you can also be a role model to yourself. Maybe not in slimming, but if you look back over your life there will almost certainly be something you did that you did well.

Can you remember a time when you made something happen? You gave up smoking, changed your job, learned to drive or made a new commitment and stuck to it. It may not have happened overnight but you hung in there until it worked. This is part of the 'being successful at anything' process. If you're prepared just to have a go, go for it. But if you think you should *give it a try*, don't bother. Saying 'I'll try' is like flying a plane from a runway that's too short. You aren't giving yourself the boost you need to get off the ground.

If you happen to be feeling so low at the moment that you can't even remember one of your past triumphs, think back to when you were a baby and you first learned to walk. Yes, that counts. You were totally motivated then. You accepted no other alternative. You pulled yourself up, you fell over, you grabbed the tablecloth and pulled that off, too. Everybody laughed at you, but you didn't care. If you'd given up on walking as easily as you've given up slimming (until now) you'd still be down on the carpet, sucking fluff.

When you think back to the things you did in your life that you were really motivated to do, you will notice that they usually involve vision plus passion plus action. And the vision is the part that comes first.

YOU GET WHAT YOU FOCUS ON

So you've decided where you're going and you've managed to get your slimming plane airborne. But human nature is a factor here, so don't expect a straight flight. You have to keep adjusting your direction and speed because of weather, other aircraft and landing conditions. But as long as you know exactly where you're going, you'll get there. Pilots don't hit a storm they didn't expect and decide to go home. They detour, they fly higher or lower, they accept that they might be delayed. But they keep going because they know where they're going.

Successful people are totally focused. And the message they are focused on is usually their own rather than somebody else's. They aren't following somebody else's dream, or somebody else's diet, or somebody else's exercise programme. And they certainly aren't focusing on what they don't want. They are aiming at what they want and trusting themselves to make the adjustments they need to make to get there.

I've been preaching this message for so long that I'm often tempted to leave it out, because to me it seems obvious. Then, just as I'm getting blasé about it, I go to a Lighten Up workshop and ask the audience what they want and they tell me they want to lose weight. And I remember that I have to keep making that point after all – because if those people had focused on being slim, they probably wouldn't need to be at the workshop. And if you had really been focused on being slim you would never have bought this book.

If you aren't getting the result you want, it's almost certainly because you aren't focusing on it. If you're still telling me you want to lose weight, I'm not surprised that you haven't.

So don't focus on being fat

When you say you want to lose weight, what do you see in your mind? Probably the weight. And the more time you spend picturing the flab you want to lose, the more energy you're investing in that image of yourself as a fat person.

It's like making a shopping list of things you don't need. You would probably get your shopping done eventually but it could take twice as long because you'd be distracted by all the things you'd decided not to buy and, of course, this is what a lot of dieters do. They walk round the supermarket with a shopping list full of salad and crispbread, but the real list is in their head and it's got everything from beer to cream cakes on it.

Give yourself a good talking to

You probably realised a few paragraphs ago that I'm going to tell you to give yourself a good talking to. If I asked you 'What do you want?' you now know that the answer is 'I want to be slimmer'. Or fitter, or healthier, or more energetic, or happier . . . anything as long as it's positive.

So isn't this just positive thinking? Well, yes it is, but positive thinking isn't the same as positive action and it shouldn't be an end in itself. It's very easy to do your positive thinking routine and nothing else. Including change.

Positive thinking is the start of the process of change, a crucial first step on the road to being slimmer, richer or anything else you fancy, but unless you take the second, third and fourth steps and keep walking, you aren't going to succeed.

Positive expectations

Positive expectations is a better way of putting it, because expectations make things happen and the most important thing that successful people have in common is their expectation that they will succeed. Non-winners don't really expect to succeed. They might hope, or wish, or try, but that doesn't count.

Sod's Law works for most people – because they expect it to. Really successful people however, know that it doesn't apply to them. Can you imagine Prince Naseem, Margaret Thatcher, Michael Jordan, the Williams sisters or Richard Branson living in the shadow of Sod's Law? They may not all be your ideal role models, but you have to admit that they know what they want, they expect to get it, and they aren't often disappointed.

SETTING GOALS

It seems that people who write down their long-term goals are much more likely to achieve them than people who don't. Goal setting has to be the most popular self-help technique ever invented, probably because it's simple and obvious. But most people still don't bother to do it.

Get it in writing

Not because you can't trust yourself, but because you may not have given all of yourself the correct instructions. You need to make sure that the message about what you really want – whether it's wealth, fame or a perfect figure – gets through to you. If you're not convinced, who else is going to be?

And there's an interesting aside here – a lot of people complain about being sabotaged by their lifestyle, family or friends when they try to lose weight. But what we've noticed is that the people who are open to sabotage are the ones who haven't really convinced themselves about what they're doing. If *you* aren't sure you're slim and glamorous, there isn't going to be much conviction in your voice when you *try* to refuse that slice of chocolate cake.

So start with long-term slimming goals and work backwards to fill in the detail on your day-to-day aspirations. Combining your short-term goals with your long-term ones will keep you moving in the right direction without getting overwhelmed.

But remember that the same golden rule applies to goal setting as it does to everything else: keep it positive. If you use negatives for goals, you'll end up telling your brain not to do anything, or worse. So if you're ready to give it a go, here's a goal-setting exercise that I've used over and over again, with slimmers, with athletes and especially with myself. It starts with asking yourself 'What do you want?' which is a question you'll be getting very familiar with over the next few weeks.

What do you want?

When you start the eight-week course you'll be doing a lot of visualising exercises like this one. They are simple and straightforward; they just take a little time and practice. There's nothing magic about them. They are a way of helping you to use your amazing brainpower purposefully instead of randomly.

Give yourself at least ten minutes to read through these questions and answer them on paper, on your computer screen or in your head. The best way of all to do it (and a lot of the other exercises in the book) is with somebody else. Then you can take it in turns to ask each other the questions without sidestepping the tricky ones.

WHAT DO YOU WANT?

Go for positive answers. Instead of writing 'I must lose weight', try something like 'I want to be slim/healthy/fit/beautiful . . .'

WHAT WILL THAT DO FOR YOU?

What benefits might you gain from whatever it is you want? Being fit, for example, might mean you can go swimming and feel good in a bikini, or wear short skirts again . . .

HOW WILL YOU KNOW THAT YOU'VE GOT WHAT YOU WANT?

What changes might happen in your life as a result of getting whatever it is that you want? Where would you be spending more time? What would you be doing that you aren't doing now?

WHAT WILL YOU SEE WHEN YOU GET WHAT YOU WANT?

This is the picture of you. What would you look like? Make it three-dimensional. Look in the mirror. What are you wearing?

WHAT WOULD YOU FEEL?

Would you glow? Would you feel warm and satisfied? Cool and in control? Happy, excited, loved, interested, glamorous, confident?

WHAT WOULD YOU HEAR?

You might hear someone special paying you a compliment, or it might just be a voice in your own head telling you how great you look. Does that ever happen? Well it could.

SEE HOW YOU WOULD LOOK, FEEL HOW YOU WOULD FEEL, IF YOU WERE THE WAY YOU WANT TO BE

Put it all together and make a movie of the new you. Give it a soundtrack. Make yourself the star. Take some time making it really convincing. Be sure it delights you.

When you've answered these questions once, I want you to get into the habit of answering them regularly. You may find that the answers change as you go through the programme. Sometimes it helps to tape the questions and play them on a Walkman or when you're alone in the car.

> *When I crash dieted, because I hadn't mentally prepared to be slimmer, my mind felt detached from my 'alien' body. The difference when I prepared my mind through visualisation from the start was that the change seemed natural, as if my mind was waiting for my body to catch up.*
>
> Sarah Tay

So you've arrived at the point where you know what you want, in quite a lot of detail. Now, all you have to do is take the decision to make the changes that will make it possible. You know what you want, you've talked yourself into it. But you still have to go out and get it.

MAKING DECISIONS

Success is a decision not an accident

So far, you've successfully lived your life, or some of it anyway, as an overweight person. You made your choice and did your fat stint and now you can take on a more challenging role.

The more clearly you can see yourself playing that new role, the easier it will be to make it happen. We'll help you by giving you the steps you need to follow, week by week in Part Two, but there are still a few preparations you need to make – so hang in a bit longer and read to the end of Part One first.

There's a flame inside all of us that can burn very brightly when we're engaged on a mission we passionately believe in – like a love affair, or fighting a war. But when we're looking at yet another slimming programme, with a history of failure behind us and the prospect of deprivation followed by more failure ahead, that flame of desire is more like a pilot light in an unused boiler.

Lighten Up will fire you up over the next eight weeks, so that you are passionate and motivated enough to succeed this time. The first step is always the hardest because change itself is challenging – and don't worry if you don't feel ready for that first step yet, that's completely normal. Our brains prefer us to stay as we are, however unhealthy or unhappy we happen to be, and if your brain is used to you sitting around a lot, watching TV and eating doughnuts, it's going to vote in favour of the status quo.

But once you get that amazing equipment you have, your body and brain, working in synchronisation you will be unstoppable. Take no notice of any initial internal protests. It may feel strange at first because doing things differently always does, but you will be making the changes that your body really wants you to make, so there isn't going to be any long-term resistance.

It's decisions not conditions that hold people back

Does any of this sound familiar?

- ★ I wish I could lose weight but I've got fat genes.
- ★ I ought to do something about it but I haven't got time.
- ★ I know I should eat a healthy diet but I have to cook for the family.
- ★ I'd love to be fitter but I can't be bothered.
- ★ I must take more exercise but I've got a really sedentary lifestyle.
- ★ I need to start working out but I'm not fit enough to exercise at the moment.
- ★ I shouldn't keep eating but I love food too much.
- ★ I wish I'd joined the health club last year but I couldn't afford it.

Well, they may sound familiar – but none of them is true.

★ Very few people have fat genes (the Pima Indians are unusual!) but even if you did have them, you can still lose weight with sensible eating and a bit of exercise.

★ Of course you can make time. Do you really need to watch three soaps a week? Couldn't you get up just half an hour earlier than you do?

★ Perhaps it might be nice for your family to eat a healthy diet as well.

★ If you really didn't care, you wouldn't have bought this book. Are you sure you can't be bothered?

★ It's easy to work some exercise into even the most sedentary lifestyle and we're going to show you how.

★ Everybody is fit enough to do at least some gentle exercise.

★ Lighten Up isn't about forcing you to hate food or stop eating, so loving food is no reason not to lose weight.

★ You don't have to pay for a health club to get some exercise. Using your body is free.

So throw away the diet and take full responsibility for the surplus weight and any other baggage you are carrying. Accepting responsibility is the magic spell that gives you the power to change.

THE CHALLENGE

Run through the 'what do you want' exercise twice before you get to Part Two. Write your answers in the Diary.

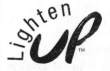

Prepare for the changes in Part Two by defining what you want and making a conscious decision to go for it.

CHAPTER EIGHT

MOTIVATION – THE FUTURE YOU

> *Are you motivated enough to Lighten Up yet?*

If you've made it this far, you've already done the toughest bit. Part One is all about thinking for yourself about what you want and what you'll do to get it. By the time you get to Chapter Nine, you will already have started the process of change.

Reading eight chapters of a book before you even get to the part you thought you bought it for takes motivation so you know what this chapter is about. Do you think you have enough motivation to complete the eight-week course in Part Two? I'm curious to know whether you're ready to make the life changes you haven't managed to make before. How do you feel about finally becoming slimmer?

THE MAGIC WORD

In the past few years I've devoted more of my time to Lighten Up than anything else, but I still do a lot of work with athletes and sportspeople, and people with all kinds of different life problems. In a single week I might see a teenager with a phobia about heights, a woman who's been trying to lose five stone for the past ten years and a boxer with training problems. Shouldn't all these people be seeing specialists? Not really, because they are already experts themselves in what's gone wrong. They can tell me at length and in great detail about the stuff that isn't working for them, and the changes they are trying to make. What they need is something new: a solution. So if you wonder what my work with a cricket team has to do with you losing weight, I can tell you – the problems may be different but the first step towards solving them is always the same: motivation.

Motivation is the modern magic word but, like positive thinking, it can be just a word. I once followed up a reference on a young man who applied for a job and I called his previous employer to get a better idea of what he was like.

'Well, he was very motivated,' she said.

'Motivated to do what?' I asked. 'What did he actually achieve while he was with you?'

'Well, not a lot, but he was very positive about everything and he never missed a day . . .'

I've met a lot of slimmers like that. They are motivated but not motivated to change. They are very enthusiastic about every new diet that appears in the bookshops and they go to at least one slimming club a week. For them, motivation isn't anything to do with changing behaviour or feeling good about themselves or eating healthy food or taking exercise; it's just a convenient substitute for action. In fact, being motivated makes it much more acceptable to go on bingeing, or slobbing out, or whatever it is they do or don't do. Because after all, they've *said* they're motivated to change, they've bought the book, they've signed up for membership, so if the diets or the slimming clubs don't work for them, it's hardly their fault. Is it?

If you want something you haven't got, you don't want it enough

These people do want to be slimmer but they don't want it enough to make it happen. They think it's going to involve such huge and complicated changes that they get overwhelmed before they start and fall back on calorie counting. And calorie counting is safe because it won't work – not for long, anyway.

Deep down, these people know they are putting off what they really want, but they allow themselves smaller and smaller bits of gratification (often chocolate-biscuit-sized) to keep them going as they delay the big payoff. We all have the same instinct to avoid pain and seek pleasure, but we short-change ourselves with short-term pleasures that lead to longer-term pain.

When you are really motivated to change you'll start to see, feel and hear the difference. True motivation doesn't keep. It has no shelf life. It either triggers immediate change or it isn't motivation. And every suggestion we'll be giving you in this chapter to help you get motivated will already be triggering the early stages of change.

CARROTS AND STICKS

How much do you know about the way you operate? People aren't born with user guides, and mostly we get by without one. But now and again it would be useful if we could just look something up instead of having to work it out every time. For example, do you know whether you're a pain avoider or a pleasure seeker? Of course we all do both, but we have our preferences; some of us will always steer clear of discomfort while others go flat out for happiness.

If you aren't sure whether you're more motivated towards or away from things, think about other people you know. It's often easier to spot these patterns in children because adults are more complex (although I sometimes think confused would be a better word), particularly if you look at how many parents and good teachers often know instinctively how to motivate children.

I promised to take a friend's children swimming one half-term and when I had a free afternoon I dropped in to collect them. My friend called her daughter, 'Hen, you've tidied your room, you can go swimming.' Her son heard the word 'swimming' and ran downstairs with his towel under his arm, only to be told, 'You're not going swimming until you've tidied your room.' I thought about it for a bit and then I asked her why she treated them differently. She didn't know, so I listened very carefully after that to see how consistent she was – and she was. When she talked to her daughter she promised treats when the homework or jobs were done, but her son was threatened with withdrawal of privileges unless he completed his tasks. It amounted to the same thing, of course, but she was unconsciously aware of her children's thought patterns and used them to generate action.

What do *you* do? Do you spend your time imagining yourself on a beach looking tanned and slender and attractive? Or do you frighten yourself with pictures of you going on holiday wearing a paisley tent? Most adults use both towards and away-from motivation to get themselves to do the things they have to do. But when it comes to doing the things they don't have to do – like losing weight – they fall back on their own personal preferences. It doesn't matter what you do, or how you do it, as long as you use your personal way of thinking to point you in the direction of success.

The big difference between Towards and Away-From Motivation is how you use it. Towards Motivation goes with thinking and speaking positively, and visualising what you want. It's a way of life – something you can do in spare moments to top up your inspiration. Away-From Motivation, on the other hand, is the short, sharp shock treatment. It's not something you dwell on, because if you do that it becomes familiar and then it's not scary any more. Away-From mmtivation is forcing yourself to look at the consequences of your actions (or inactions) once in a while. Just so that you know what's out there.

Towards Motivation

Of course, we've already talked about Towards Motivation. When we make positive statements about what we want and visualise a brighter future for ourselves, we're generating our own Towards Motivation.

Desperation motivation

Towards mmtivation is powerful, easy to nurture and develop, and we suggest you make it a permanent part of your life. But

Away-From Motivation is a force to be reckoned with as well. We sometimes make the most drastic changes in our lives when we get really scared. Working as a personal trainer I used to meet a lot of people who started exercising after their first heart attack or went into training five nights a week when they were dropped from a team. And the sports world is full of men and women who used a poor start in life to motivate them away from pain and poverty, and into personal success.

Away-From Motivation comes with a health warning – **Take in very small doses once in a blue moon**.

The power of pain

Do you ever hear a voice in your head nagging you about the washing up, just as you're relaxing after dinner? And as you're about to drag yourself into the kitchen, another voice chips in and says, 'Hang on, you might as well watch the end of the news, the dishes can wait.' Or maybe that sort of commentary comes with your paperwork, or your ironing, or cleaning the car.

And what about all the other things you've been meaning to do for so long? What keeps you from making a dynamic career change? Why don't you get your overdraft sorted? Isn't it time you had a night off the beer? Shouldn't you be eating more fruit and veggies? Why is it so long since you got your bike out?

You know very well that activating your own particular 'I wish' list would improve your quality of life if you could only bring yourself to do it. But you don't. Why? Because you just aren't motivated enough.

Chances are that you're a creature of comfort like everybody else. You get a lot of pleasure from not taking any of those positive, healthy, enterprising actions. If you don't upgrade your job, you keep the undemanding one and avoid the pressure. If you don't drink less beer you can spend more time at the pub. If you stick with the escalating overdraft you can go on buying cars you can't afford. If you don't bother with a healthy diet you can go on enjoying the fast food. And so on.

Your current lifestyle may not be doing you much good, but it's comfortable and familiar. For most people the fear of losing something or giving something up – even a glass of wine or an extra hour in bed – is much stronger than the excitement of doing something new, like going to the gym after work or getting up early enough for a morning jog. That's understandable. We can't actually experience the future so we work hard to hang on to the present that we can see, touch, hear and smell. The present has to get pretty uncomfortable before we are going to be willing to change it, but you can speed up the process.

Flabbergasted, flab'ér-gästed *(coll.):*
feeling of horror when you look in the mirror
and realise how much weight you have gained

Breaking the pain barrier is a great motivator for making positive life changes. Sometimes nothing will shift a pattern of continuous dysfunctional behaviour until the person who owns that behaviour reaches their personal threshold of discomfort – or pain. It's for you to decide whether this particular reaction – or strategy – will work for you. Do you need to get to the point where you wake up in the morning and can't look at yourself in the mirror because it's just too painful? Are you at that point already?

If you aren't sure, get out your photo album and look at some holiday pictures from five or ten years ago. Or try on some clothes that have been in the back of the wardrobe for way too long. Don't dwell on it. Do it and get back to your long-term strategy – focusing on what you actually want.

The success system

So do you usually back away from things you don't like? Or are you drawn to what you want? Or both? Working with the way you are is great, but the more options and strategies you can use, the more chance of success you will have. So see if you can motivate yourself both ways.

Lighten Up helps you build your own success system by putting maximum pressure behind you to change as well as a compelling vision in front to move you forward.

When I used to teach aerobics I got frustrated with the minimal effort that most of the class put into the movements.

Eventually (like every other aerobics teacher, I suppose) I found that whatever I was demonstrating got scaled down by the class, so in order to keep them exercising at a reasonable level I had to make huge exaggerated movements myself. It was like cranking them up physically. The Lighten Up process shows you how to do exactly the same thing for yourself psychologically.

SEEING THE FUTURE

The next most important motivation-generating tool is visualisation. And visualisation, like positive thinking, is one of those self-help methods that has been around so long that it's misunderstood and undervalued.

The eight-week course you're about to start will use your visualisation skills extensively. And if you think you can't make pictures in your mind, just stop for a minute and picture your front door. We all think in pictures, but some people have managed to fine-tune it so that they think in full technicolour with surround sound and smell and touch thrown in. *And* they have a volume switch as well as an on/off button.

So don't be fooled by the word visualisation; there's much more to it than meets the eye. You will be using all five of your senses – or six, if you're gifted that way.

Turn your life around

When a person comes along and says to us, 'I'm fed up with this and I really think I ought to do something about it,' we immediately know that nothing's going to happen until we can get him (or her) to say, 'I can't go on like this, I'm making some changes – and I don't care what it takes, I'm ready to do it.' That tells us that they've been through the away-from motivation process and they are looking for a way forward.

So how do we get somebody to change from the first statement to the second? Simply by making the future seem as real as the present. And all it takes is a little imagination and a lot of practice.

Practice

Practice is the secret of making visualisation work for you, which is why this powerful life-changing tool isn't used as much as it could be. Most people think that visualisation is more to do with inspiration than perspiration when, in fact, out of all the techniques we teach, it's probably the one that needs most repetition to make it really effective. (You'll notice we said repetition, we didn't say hard work.)

If you look at the faces of athletes just before a competition, chances are they're seeing themselves winning, hearing the crowd and feeling the ground under their feet, over and over again. Or, at least, that's what the successful ones are doing. The less successful ones are using the visualisation process – or rather letting it use them – to make them feel bad. They are picturing their last bad shot, or their last fall, or the last opponent who beat them. Visualisation is a double-edged sword and the key to making it work for you is to keep doing it until it's totally under your control.

Some athletes I've worked with recently have been to see me, run through a couple of visualisation exercises and gone away again, convinced that they'd bought the magic formula and that one dose was enough. But, in fact, visualisation is more like antibiotics – you need to take the whole course before your own immune system kicks in again and keeps you going.

A QUICK VISUALISATION EXERCISE

Think of the last really great holiday you had. Remember some of the things you saw, and heard and felt, the sky, the scenery, the people you were with and the food you ate, and make it as close and bright and clear as you can. As you relive the experience for a few seconds, you'll get a glimmer of the good feelings you had at the time.

Now imagine your next holiday. The one you haven't had yet, in the place you've always wanted to visit. Can you

continued

---

lose yourself in a picture out of one of the brochures? Can you feel the sun or the breeze or the sea and hear the sounds around you?

The interesting thing about this is that your brain doesn't know the difference between the real holiday and the one you made up – and you can use this to your advantage. After all, if you can visualise yourself on a holiday that never happened, how much easier will it be to see yourself looking slim and wonderful. You may even have seen yourself looking that way in the not too distant past.

We assume you're reading this book because you think you would like to lose weight. Well, take the first step now. Turn that thought into a positive statement and imagine yourself looking as slim as you would like to be. As we said before, you'll eventually get what you focus on so make sure you are focusing on what you want. Get a really clear picture of how different you'll look – will your face change shape? Will you get a new haircut to suit your new image? What will your clothes be like? Are you going to start wearing more fitted tops to show off your trim waist and a flat stomach? Summery, spaghetti-strap dresses to reveal your fat-free arms? Shorter skirts to emphasise your shapely legs? Really *see* your new self.

You've probably got the message by now. Just think how useful it will be when your brain is at your disposal rather than randomly trying to make you happy by suggesting you need an ice-cream when you really need to go for a walk. Wouldn't it be great if you could control your feelings, rather than letting your feelings order you to have a snack every time there's a crisis? Wouldn't it be great if you could control your own emotions and make your own decisions about what you wanted to do and eat and feel, and how you wanted to look?

Lighten Up encourages you to build up some visualising muscle so that you can use it to direct your thoughts and actions wherever you want.

Bah, humbug!

Do you remember the *Christmas Carol* story? Scrooge changes when the Spirit of Christmas Future shows him what his life will be like if he hangs on to his wealth instead of taking the risk of sharing it with other people, making friends and having fun. It's not until the pain level is raised to the point where the old man is reduced to tears that he's willing to let go of everything he's got and take a chance on a happier future.

Try this yourself at home

ANOTHER VISUALISATION EXERCISE

Think of yourself as you are now, the way you look and the way you feel at this moment and then think what you would like to change. You can do this by yourself, sitting just as you are, with the book on your lap, but you'll get more out of it if you stand up and get someone else to read it to you.

Give yourself ten minutes to answer these questions:

★ If I go on as I am now (eating too much, eating the wrong things, sitting down too much, drinking . . .) what will my life be like six months from now?

★ Don't just use words: 'I'll have trouble getting upstairs, my relationship will be finished, the children will be ashamed of me, my health will suffer . . .' Make it a colour movie and put as much feeling into it as you can stand. Then step right into yourself and get a feel for what your life will be like if your current lifestyle continues.

★ Now ask yourself the same question again. This time travel not just six months ahead but a whole year. See yourself, hear yourself and feel what it would be like to be you – the way you'll be if you carry on with your current lifestyle.

continued

> ★ Repeat the process three more times, going two years
> and then five years into the future and, finally, taking a
> giant leap into your next decade. Look at what you've
> become.
>
> When you've had as much as you can stand of that grim
> future, take a deep breath and turn the situation around.
> Run through the same questions again, but, this time, see
> yourself the way you will be if you do things differently.
> What will you look and feel like in five years' time if you
> make those changes you want to make right now? Just think
> how great you are going to feel when you've turned your life
> around.

Are you motivated yet? Because if you aren't, just keep
repeating this exercise over and over again until it works.

THE LAST WORD IN DECISION MAKING

Are you ready yet? Of course, we're assuming that you actually
made your decision back in Chapter Seven to be slimmer, fitter
and healthier for ever, but how do you know it's a decision, not
a wish?

When I worked for a health club, the same people used to
join, drop out, rejoin and drop out over and over again. The first
time I came across this was with a young woman who joined up
in September to get rid of the after-effects of too much tapas and
paella on her summer holiday. She hung in until November, disappeared for a while, then phoned in December to let me know
she wouldn't be coming in again.

'What happened? I asked, 'did you lose the weight already
just by thinking about it?'

'No,' she said, 'it's just that with the office party next week
and all the pre-Christmas celebrations, there doesn't seem to
be much point in a lot of self-denial while everybody else is
having fun.'

'Who said anything about self-denial?' I argued – but I could not change her mind.

'I'll be back in the New Year,' she told me. 'I know I really must try to get back in shape.'

As I've said before, when I hear words like 'try' and 'must' and 'have to', warning bells ring in my head. More about that in a minute, though.

True to her word, she turned up again in January and she wasn't the only one. There's always a big membership surge at that time of year, and it's not because everybody suddenly feels full of energy and vitality. It's because, after the Christmas ritual of over-indulgence, lots of us still feel that we have to follow up with a period of penance and self-denial. But it's just a ritual. It doesn't mean anything, so it doesn't usually last. After two or three weeks of pain, discomfort and inconvenience, we figure we've paid for the fun we had and get right back into sitting in the car, in the office, and in front of the TV.

Conscience money

When I first started to work in the fitness industry I was amazed at how many people signed up for a year's membership at vast expense and then disappeared before they got their money's worth. What I didn't realise was that membership fees for some of them was like paying a fine for bad behaviour. It was a gesture they made to prove they were sorry for their past excesses – but they weren't prepared to put in the energy, time and effort as well. Just the money.

Unfortunately, money doesn't make you thin (in spite of what the liposuction and fat pill industries would have us believe). There's still no satisfactory substitute for plenty of exercise and healthy eating. All money can do is salve your conscience for a while.

How do they do that?

But what about the people who get up on 1 January, look at themselves in the mirror, say 'time to change' and then do it?

They are the people who pay their club membership and get the last drop of value out of it. Or maybe they don't even join a club. Instead, they get up an hour earlier, right through the cold dark mornings of January, February and March, and go for a run. Perhaps they just sell their car and buy a bike. Whatever it is they do, they do it regularly and it becomes part of their routine, part of their life, even part of who they are.

Being childish

These people fall into two groups. One group never got out of the childish habit of being active and eating when they were hungry. And the other group relearned that habit all over again. I'm lucky because I'm one of the first group who never grew up. I've always loved exercise, it makes me feel good while I'm doing it and even better afterwards. When I first started work in the fitness industry, it was a shock to me to realise that not all my clients felt the same. Once I understood that lots of people found exercise hard, painful and boring, I wasn't surprised they couldn't keep it up for long. You might put your hand on a hot stove once, but you don't leave it there if you've got any sense. In fact, I'm much more surprised that people who hate exercising manage to hang in with it for as long as some of them do.

So I decided that it must be possible to help that second group of people who were battling against all those habits of inactivity and unhealthy eating. And I knew it wouldn't be too difficult because most people, like the lady who dropped out and dropped in again, are halfway there already. They *know* deep down what's good for them – otherwise they wouldn't decide to lead a more active life and eat healthier food every January (even if they do abandon the idea by March).

But of course, knowing's not enough. It's doing that makes the difference. And this is where we stop talking about Lighten Up and start doing it.

THE CHALLENGE

Top up your Towards Motivation: take exactly ten minutes and make a huge list in your Diary of what you would get out of being slimmer, fitter and healthier. There should be at least twenty items on the list and, if you have time, go for more.

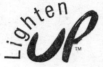 *You can be as slim as you want to be if you're motivated enough. And if you're not sure whether you are ready to start the Lighten Up programme, here's what you do:*

Look at the carrots and sticks in your life – whatever is driving you away from your current lifestyle and drawing you to be slimmer, fitter and healthier. Get in touch with your own motivation.

Spend some time visualising both what you want and what you don't want, and use the power of your imagination to strengthen those images. See if you can make those forces stronger and more irresistible.

PART

After my first couple of weeks of Lightening Up, I started to feel much better in myself. It was so great to be losing weight and eating properly for a change. Once I could see and feel the pounds coming off that encouraged me even more and all the techniques soon became second nature to me.

Lighten Up gently introduced exercise and before long I was doing it without even thinking about it. I never used to exercise at all before and now it's part of my life. It's also made me realise the importance of eating the right foods and the effect they have on the way you feel. In fact, I've made a complete lifestyle change! I make sure I allocate an hour each day for exercise if possible, eat lots of fruit and really think about what I would like to eat as opposed to just grabbing anything.

I feel a lot more in control of myself now – if I want to have wine, or cake or whatever I will, but I know it is all about balance and moderation, and I know when to stop.

I don't have to worry about putting weight back on because the changes I've made are part of my lifestyle now – I don't have to think about them or struggle with them. Best of all, I feel absolutely brilliant, full of energy, healthy, confident and optimistic.

Nicola Brown

THE EIGHT-WEEK COURSE

Before you start

It's time to put all those memories of failed weight loss attempts behind you and leave all your preconceptions of what makes a successful slimming programme at the door. The Lighten Up course is going to be unlike anything you've ever tried before – and, unlike everything else you've tried before, it works! Lighten Up is not a diet. You won't be starving yourself or counting calories – in fact we don't even talk about nutrition in detail until Chapter Twelve. Instead you're going to spend the first few weeks of the programme sorting out your mind and getting to know your current behaviour patterns. This may sound radical – and you probably can't see how this could possibly help you – but you're just going to have to trust us on this one: the Lighten Up programme works.

> *My attitude has been transformed, permanently in my opinion. The change in my eating has also been astonishing. The most amazing thing about all of this is just how much I've enjoyed the process. From the day of the workshop I've felt enthusiastic and motivated, knowing I'll reach my goal.*
>
> Jamie Smart

Our Winter 2000 survey gave a 68 per cent success rate for the Lighten Up programme and *all* the people who lost weight felt, like Jamie, that they had made a permanent change. This compares with a generally accepted 5 per cent average success rate for all other slimming programmes.

The aim of the Lighten Up Eight-week Course is to put you in control of your weight, and give you everything you need to become as slim as you want to be. However, please remember, it is an *eight-week* course so if, at the end of week one or two (or even three) we still haven't covered a topic you think is important, don't panic. The chances are it'll be coming up in the next week or so. And we promise that by the end of the eight weeks you'll have all you need to help you become slimmer, fitter and healthier.

The Lighten Up programme

Decide which day your new week is going to begin and then set aside some time the day before to sit quietly by yourself, read the next chapter and look through the exercises for the first time. This will give you an idea of what you'll be doing during the week and then you can plan two or three 'time out' periods to re-visit the chapter, doing the exercises as you go along.

If you have a busy or a difficult week – or even a disastrous one – for any reason, just start the chapter over again. And, whether you're doing a particular week for the first or even the third time, always make sure you are sitting down comfortably without any interruptions or distractions. The Lighten Up programme works much better when you are relaxed and focused on what you are doing.

You'll come across some exercises headed 'Do this now', which you can easily do as you go along. They are fun and they'll give you a clear idea of where you are at the moment, and how much you're changing.

Towards the end of each section you'll find the Lighten Up Challenges and instructions for the week. These are the things we'll be asking you to focus on and incorporate into your daily life, and they'll range from positive visualisations to ways to curb food cravings and get more exercise. At the very end you'll find a checklist, which will make crystal clear what you need to do every day. Photocopy this seven times, stick it in your diary entry for each day of the week and cross the items off as you do them.

Each week, you'll be focusing on these three areas of your life:

★ Your eating habits – how to know when you're genuinely hungry and enjoy a more healthy, balanced diet.
★ Your self-image – yes you really can believe in yourself as a slim, fit and active person and live the lifestyle that fits the dream.
★ Your activity levels – you'll be encouraged to include more regular, comfortable exercise in your daily routine.

CHAPTER NINE

WEEK ONE
OF THE
EIGHT-WEEK
COURSE

THE SUCCESSFUL SLIMMING FORMULA

> *When you look in the mirror, you are looking at the problem.*
> *But remember, you are also looking at the solution.*

Why aren't you a successful slimmer yet?

Most people want to succeed, whether in business, life or losing weight. So why do so few of us actually manage it? The success rate when it comes to slimming is only 5 per cent, so anyone who's already tried to lose weight and failed is in a strong majority. But despite the odds, the answer to this question is actually very simple: the people who don't succeed in slimming (or anything else) are using the wrong formula. Yes, there really is a 'successful slimming' formula. It's taken ten years to research and test, but here it is, set out step by step in the Lighten Up eight-week programme.

When I first became interested in slimming, I made it my mission to talk to as many successful slimmers as I could find. I wanted to know how they had succeeded where the other 95 per cent had failed.

What I discovered is that the successful slimmers were the ones who had made permanent changes to their lifestyle. The first thing they altered was their attitude to eating, exercise and life in general, followed by their habits – and quite small habits were often enough to make a big difference. I remember one woman who decided to walk her children to school every day instead of driving them. It was a mile each way, so she was doing four miles a day and that simple life change was enough, over a six-month period, to help her lose all the weight she wanted. It was good for the children too – although, of course, they only walked half the distance. The remarkable thing about this lady is not the fact that she discovered she could easily walk four miles a day; it was the way in which she made the decision to do it and then stuck to that decision.

The exciting thing about all the successful slimmers we meet is that they *all* use similar techniques to help themselves make the necessary decisions and changes. And these are the techniques we're going to teach you over the next eight weeks.

But there's one very important point. The difference between a successful slimmer and a failed one has nothing to do with luck, dieting or having a high metabolic rate. It all comes down to how much you want to change. And once you really start to change you'll find you won't ever want to turn back.

We follow up all the people who come on the Lighten Up courses (if they want us to) and hear some inspiring stories. Recently I spoke to one lady who said 'Well, I've lost twenty thousand pounds.'

'Don't you think that's a bit much?' I asked her.

'If it hadn't been for Lighten Up,' she said, 'I wouldn't have bought this horse.'

She had won a lot of prizes when she was younger, but for the past twenty years her weight had stopped her riding – among other things. 'Now that I'm slim enough to ride again,' she added, 'I'm having far too much fun to go back to my old lifestyle.'

We don't expect many people to start show jumping as a result of Lightening Up. The key word in this story is not 'horse' but 'fun'. Fun is going to mean different things to different people – but whether you want to wear a bikini, learn to tango or join your local rugby team, we want you to be slim, fit and healthy enough to do it.

So now that you're ready to start, it's important that you take the programme one week at a time, be as open as possible to all the ideas and do the various exercises as they come along. Some of them will work better for you than others, but you won't know which until you give them a try. It's taken ten years to get this programme into the shape and pace that works best, so don't analyse or personalise or pick and mix. Just do it all and see what happens – you'll find you surprise yourself.

However, please bear in mind that you aren't going to end up doing *anything* for life just because we tell you to. One of our original Lighten Uppers complained after a few weeks that he couldn't cope with healthy eating. When we asked him what he meant it turned out that he'd forced himself to eat carrots (which he'd always hated) every day for two weeks before giving up completely and going back to his original high-fat, low-fit eating habits. 'You said carrots were good for us,' he complained.

The success of the Lighten Up programme doesn't depend on you following rigid rules. We don't expect you to eat or do anything you don't like. We're just asking you to give it all a go. You can keep the best and delete the rest when you know yourself a little better.

Are you ready?

★ Each week we'll give you some new things to think about and some other things to do. Week One is much more about thinking than doing, but bear with us as it's vital to get your brain into gear before you engage your body.

★ Each week, as we go through the programme, try out all the techniques and ideas as they are introduced. Do them all. The Lighten Up Diary and Challenges at the end of each chapter will then summarise everything we've worked on this week and suggest what you should focus on and be doing on a daily basis for the rest of the week.

★ You already have a notebook and we're hoping you're already in the habit of using it so it will be easy to start your Lighten Up Diary.

★ You might like to recruit a supportive friend as a lot of the exercises work very well if you have someone to ask you the questions and give you feedback. Of course it's even better if your friend wants to be slimmer as well – that way you can take it in turns and give each other some support and encouragement.

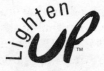 **WEEK ONE**

In Week One we'll be introducing you to some of the simplest and most powerful Lighten Up techniques.

★ Exercise Your Right to Pleasure: associating pain with an inactive lifestyle and pleasure with a healthy one.
★ Mind your Language: you can if you think you can.
★ The Pleasure of Eating: the pain and pleasure principle applied to eating.
★ Think Thin: creating a vision of how you want to be, which is so powerful and compelling that you're drawn towards it.
★ Measure Your Success: monitoring your progress without weighing yourself.
★ Be Your Own Role Model: learning to trust yourself and make your own decisions.
★ The Power of Decisions: taking control of your own life by making a decision and signing a contract.
★ The Lighten Up Diary: your personal support system for the next eight weeks.

EXERCISE YOUR RIGHT TO PLEASURE

This is the first step of the Lighten Up programme. How long have you been sitting down, reading this? Ten minutes? Half an hour? Whatever the answer, when you have read to the end of this section put the book down, stretch, take a walk around the block and come back to it.

DO THIS NOW Remember the list of words in Chapter Six? Turn back to it for a moment. Which words do you associate with exercise? Some people get an adrenaline surge just by thinking about going for a swim or a run or a step class. But a lot of people don't.

A lot of people hate the idea of exercise. They think it's going to hurt. They know they are going to be miserable and they set out to prove themselves right.

Expecting it to be hell, people often start a new slimming programme by exercising daily at way above their personal limits, usually doing something they dislike but think is good for them – like going to the gym – rather than something they might find enjoyable – like taking a dance class. And so the self-fulfilling prophecy strikes again. After a few weeks of painful workouts, it's no wonder they often go back to the pleasures they miss, the comfort they've denied themselves and a happy, lardy life.

Everything we do is decided by whether we think our actions will lead to pleasure or pain. We have an internal biological mechanism that constantly seeks to avoid pain and find pleasure, but the problem is that this mechanism works best in the short term. If you want to be slim, fit and happy in the long term, you need to engage your brain. Maybe you never associated exercise with pleasure before – it's easy to go for the much quicker fix and sit down instead with a biscuit and a cup of tea. But if you know you want a fitter, slimmer, healthier future, Lighten Up can help you re-motivate yourself towards attaining long-term future pleasure, so that you don't keep giving up and sitting down. And you can start this process off straight away by thinking about the pleasure you'll get from being slimmer, fitter and healthier.

DO THIS NOW Now, it's time for you to stop reading and take that short, brisk walk. If you hear yourself saying: 'I can't, I haven't got time, it's raining, I'm tired . . . ', just tell yourself to shut up. Think about how good you'll feel when you're actually walking and how wonderful you'll feel when go to bed tonight with a relaxed body and a relaxed mind.

If your body lets you down, get your mind to fill in the blanks

If you can't get up and get out right now for some good reason – you have a knee injury perhaps, or you have flu, or you're on a train or a plane, do some deep breathing instead and *imagine* yourself taking that walk. Alan Davies, the rugby coach, tells the story of how, after the car crash that nearly killed him, he spent months in hospital, in plaster and almost immobilised. During that time he exercised, every day, in his mind following the exercise routine he used when he was playing rugby himself. He jogged, he worked out and he lifted weights – in his head. Whenever possible he contracted the muscles he would have been using if this had been a real, physical training session. When he finally left hospital, the doctors and physiotherapists were amazed at how quickly he regained his strength and returned to his usual high levels of activity.

So no excuses. If you can't do it, imagine you can. Take the first steps in your mind and, sooner than you think, you'll be putting on your walking shoes and heading out of the door.

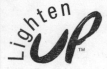

Every time you find yourself sitting down for more than half an hour take a break, have a stretch and walk for a few minutes. Keep doing this for the rest of the week.

MIND YOUR LANGUAGE

We've already been dropping hints about the way you talk to yourself (let's face it, everybody does it, so you might as well do it constructively) and now it's time to experiment. Are you *expecting* to be slimmer by the end of this book, or are you just *hoping* you will be?

Do you remember when you were at school, the adults in your life were constantly telling you all the things you should be doing and all the things you ought not to be doing. Didn't that make you feel rebellious? So why are you still using that kind of language when you talk to yourself?

 Get your pen and write down the answers – either right here in the book or in your Lighten Up Diary.

Self-abuse

★ What is it that you want to be? Is it slimmer, healthier, fitter, more comfortable with yourself? Write down your answer (not a whole sentence, just what you'd like to be):

....

★ When you've written down your objective, close your eyes and say, 'I *should* be ....'

★ What sort of image do you see when you say that to yourself? Do you get a picture, or just some words? Is it clear, or dim and indistinct? Whatever it is, write it down:

....

....

★ How do you *feel* when you say to yourself 'I *should* be ....'? Do you feel positive and optimistic, or doubtful, or anything in between?

....

Now, repeat this exercise another **six** times. Each time you will phrase what you want slightly differently, but afterwards you'll ask yourself the same question:
'I *hope* I'll be ....'

★ Write down the image you get when you say that:

....

....

★ How did you *feel* when you said 'I *hope* I'll be ....'?

....

'I *could* be ....'

★ Write down the image you get when you say that:

....

....

★ How did you *feel* when you said 'I *could* be ....'?

_____

'I *need* to be ....'

★ Write down the image you get when you say that:

....

....

★ How did you *feel* when you said 'I *need* to be ....'?

....

'I *might* be ....'

★ Write down the image you get when you say that:

....

....

★ How did you *feel* when you said 'I *might* be ....'?

....

'I *have* to be ....'

★ Write down the image you get when you say that:

....

....

★ How did you *feel* when you said 'I *have* to be ....'?

....

'I *ought* to be ....'

★ Write down the image you get when you say that:

....

....

★ How did you *feel* when you said 'I *ought* to be ....'?

....

Now let's ask nicely

Think about what you want again, but this time, imagine that you *really expect* it to happen.

'I *will* be ....'

★ Write down the image you get when you say that:

....

....

★ How did you *feel* when you said 'I *will* be ....'?

....

'I *want* to be ....'

★ Write down the image you get when you say that:

....

....

★ How did you *feel* when you said 'I *want* to be.....................'?

....

'I *am going* to be ....'

★ Write down the image you get when you say that:

....

....

★ How did you *feel* when you said 'I *am going* to be ....'?

....

'I *expect* to be ....'

★ Write down the image you get when you say that:

....

....

★ How did you *feel* when you said 'I *expect* to be ....'?

....

It doesn't matter whether you believe what you're saying or not – though the chances are that, at first, you'll believe the first set of statements more readily than the second. Just say the words and write down how the words make you feel.

If you want to get results, *hoping* is never good enough. *Expecting* gets results. Don't leave the things you really want to chance: '*It might happen, it could happen . . .*' Those statements have doubt built into them.

Your brain believes what you tell it, so it's time you gave it some more encouraging words. We've seen a lot of promising athletes telling themselves they couldn't do something and then proving themselves right. Some of those athletes have had very short careers. What a contrast with champions like Pete Sampras and Tiger Woods, who would never, in a thousand years, tell themselves they couldn't win.

In this media-frenzied world we're bombarded with messages from all directions telling us how we should look, what our goals ought to be, how we should judge ourselves. It's time for you to take control of this input and give yourself some positive messages for a change. And that's what this exercise is all about.

Remember: You can if you think you can.

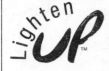 Repeat this exercise as often as you like. But if you've finished with it for now, before you turn the page, just mark the statement that gives you the best feeling.

THE PLEASURE OF EATING

The pain and pleasure principle applies to eating just as much as to exercise. The reason that we always start the eight-week programme by talking about exercise is simply because what you do in terms of exercise is more important than what you eat when you want to lose weight.

A lot of people just don't like the idea of exercise. It's that simple. But the relationship most slimmers have with food tends to be much more complicated. A lot of people see food as their enemy – and this was a shock to me at first, because I enjoy eating and cooking and sharing meals. For me food is one of life's great pleasures.

Given the love-hate relationship so many people have with food, we believe it's very important that one of your first aims as a slimmer should be to learn how to enjoy eating again. We've noticed that most people who worry about their weight eat quickly and guiltily. They don't dare take time to taste what they eat – which is why they often go for extreme tastes like very sweet or very salty snacks. While the food's in their mouths they feel relief from the craving – but not much sensual pleasure.

HOW MUCH OF WHAT YOU DON'T WANT IS ENOUGH?

People who eat too much are eating for reasons other than hunger and are therefore trying to fill a bottomless hole. You can't ever satisfy a longing for self-esteem, or love or happiness with a piece of chocolate cake, though you might get some temporary comfort from it.

If you could actually enjoy the food you ate, wouldn't that make a difference to the way you ate it? Wouldn't you feel more like slowing down and really tasting each delicious mouthful? And eating like this might even make you feel full much sooner than you usually do.

The Lighten Up message for both eating and exercise is the same: **Enjoy**.

If you enjoy what you do and what you eat, you're much more likely to choose the healthy food that your body needs and take the right amount of exercise for you.

MAKING THE BREAK

If you speak to the 68 per cent of people who have lost weight on the Lighten Up programme and kept it off, they'll probably tell you that the thought of eating well and exercising regularly used to be painful to them – until, one day they turned their attitudes around. *Now* they find the thought of endless chips and chocolate less appealing because they know how fat and overfull they are going to feel after they've eaten them. This successful 68 per cent have also learned to enjoy being active and they hate the thought of missing out on exercise. They've made it part of their daily routine.

HOW DID THEY DO THAT?

By doing what we will be doing over the next eight weeks and *changing the way they think as well as what they do and what they eat.*

THINK THIN

You've heard the saying: *You are what you eat* . . . well, here's a better one: *You are what you think.*

Our lives are governed by our thoughts and if you think you are fat and overweight, you'll have pictures in your mind which support this. You will be building your daily life on this image – reinforcing the belief that you are fat every time you think about it. Conventional diets don't deal with people's thoughts. Maybe that's another reason why so many people regain all their weight again so soon after a diet. They still *think* they're fat. They don't know how to live thin. And slowly the weight creeps back on to wherever they've convinced themselves it belongs.

The next exercise, the Open Door, will help you develop an even clearer positive image of yourself. Each and every time you do it you are sending a message to your unconscious mind, which reminds you, right now, that you are losing weight.

The Open Door focuses your mind on your goal, making it more powerful and real. It helps to make you aware that each time you say 'no' to food when you're not hungry, you're saying 'yes' to being slimmer and moving closer to your future self. The more real the image, the less negative and judgemental you will be. You'll be turning automatically towards a stronger sense of yourself as you want to be.

Thinking thin is a cliché. And it works. If it hasn't worked for you before, there could be two reasons: either you didn't believe it or you didn't do it often enough. It's as simple as that.

The Open Door (with thanks to Paul McKenna)

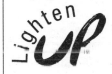
The Open Door is a visualisation exercise. You know you can do it, because you already did a similar one in Chapter Eight when, like Scrooge, you looked at your future and your past.

Athletes use visualisation to achieve the most amazing results. You can use it to make you run faster, lose weight or achieve your life's ambitions. Sounds too easy? Well actually, that's the catch. It's easy to do – everybody can daydream – but, if you want real results, you have to be prepared to go into mental training and put in plenty of practice.

DO THIS NOW You can do this alone, or with a friend reading out the instructions to you. Or you could buy the Lighten Up cassette which will talk you through the main Lighten Up visualisation exercises. Find a place where you won't be disturbed for at least ten minutes and read this aloud a couple of times before you do it yourself. The best way is to imagine that you are giving the instructions to somebody else. Make it somebody you know well so that you can really picture them doing it.

1 Stand up with a couple of feet of space in front of you.
2 Close your eyes and see your front door in your mind. Make it a life-size image and imagine you are standing outside, watching it open.
3 Now imagine, as your door opens in front of you, that there is an image of you at some time in the future, standing there in the hallway.
4 That image of the future you is slimmer, fitter and healthier. See yourself exactly as you want to be. You are at your ideal weight, glowing with health and feeling confident and happy.
5 Make the picture life-size and notice the firmness and clarity of your skin, the muscle and tone of your body.
6 Make the picture so clear and bright that you could reach out and touch it. Make it vivid, colourful and brilliant. It doesn't matter if it's not as sharp as you want it at first because, with daily practice, your image will become more real.
7 Now imagine the future you turning right round so that you can see yourself from every angle.
8 When the future you has turned right round and is facing away from you again, step forward into yourself. Literally walk into your new, slim, fit and healthy body, like putting on a new skin. Always walk into your back view. Don't try to walk into yourself face to face, it's too weird.
9 As you do this, notice how it feels, notice how light and elegant you've become. Feel the comfort and grace of your movements as you begin to open your eyes in the new you.
10 Pause for a moment and recognise how this changes the way you feel.

11 Take that feeling and run through the exercise again. This time double the power, make it crystal clear, and see how attractive you look and feel as your confidence increases.

Once you've read through this exercise a couple of times, as if you were talking somebody else through it, the next thing to do is to talk *yourself* through it. Sit, just as you are, looking at the page. Read each instruction aloud to yourself and then pause for a moment with your eyes closed and wait for the pictures (or feelings, or sounds) to come. Once you can see everything clearly, move on to the next instruction until you have reached number 11.

If it helps, you could record yourself reading the instructions and then play the tape instead of reading out of the book.

Many people see themselves as they were in the past or as they are in the present when they do this exercise. It may be difficult at first to picture the future you because it's not something you often think about. So make sure you are looking into the future and not dwelling on the past. You may never have seen yourself looking like this – or, at least, not for a long time. So use your imagination to see what you would like to see.

We all think in pictures and dream in pictures, so we can all go through the Open Door. It may take a little longer for some people to do it consciously whenever they want to, but with a little practice it will become second nature.

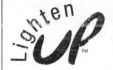

Repeat this exercise every day as you come closer and closer to becoming the future you right now.

MEASURE YOUR SUCCESS

The Open Door exercise is designed to help you focus on what you want. So, next time we ask you what you want you should be able to describe it in quite a lot of detail. The image of yourself as you want to be should now be much clearer and so long as you hold this picture in your mind you'll have all the will-power you need to succeed. You won't need to struggle with sensible eating or force yourself to be more active. The positive actions you're taking will move you closer to the glowing, slimmer, future you.

In the early days of Lighten Up, people would queue up for the weigh-in they assumed was going to happen at the beginning of a workshop. So I used to tell them the story of my friend Lisa, who deliberately left her scales behind when she moved flats – she couldn't quite bring herself to throw them out. A week later, the girl who took over her old place called round to see her. She had a couple of pot plants and the scales in a carrier bag. 'You left these behind,' she said. 'Oh, and by the way, those scales are totally inaccurate, they're all over the place, I nearly threw them out – but you don't need to weigh yourself anyway, do you?'

Lisa told me the story herself, then she said, 'I feel so cross about all those bad days I had when I'd gained a couple of pounds. I remember thinking my weight was fluctuating a lot.' Then she looked at me and shook her head. 'Don't even think about saying it.'

'I told you so,' I said.

Scales are a slimmer's worst enemy and, even if you have ones that work, remember that they aren't just weighing fat. They're weighing everything else as well: muscle, bone, skin and water, but although most people don't in theory mind increasing muscle and bone density they'll still worry about it when it shows up on the scales. Of course, you can now get high-tech scales that pass an electrical impulse through your body to assess how much fat you're carrying but we still don't advise you to look at yourself in that kind of day-to-day detail. Relying on scales for feedback just chips away at your self-belief. If you feel you have to get on the scales every day, you'll find it harder to trust some of the basic Lighten Up techniques you'll be using over the next few weeks, like the Hunger Scale and Think Before You Eat.

There's also a lot more to slimming than shedding fat. If you just shed fat, it's very likely to creep back on again. If you want to be permanently slimmer you'll have to replace some of that fat with energy-burning muscle. Fat takes up to five times more space on your body than muscle, but muscle weighs a lot more so the scales *won't* show that rapid reduction you've been hoping for.

A person's weight can also fluctuate from day to day for many biological reasons – and women, in particular, retain more fluid at some times of the month than at others. More important, even with modern scales it's hard to be exact about your muscle mass and tone, or work out exactly what proportion of your weight is made up of fat, muscle or bone. Over the years, Lighten Up has seen hundreds of people who couldn't understand why their jeans were getting baggier when the scales didn't register any change for three, four, five, or even six weeks. The reason, of course, was that as they were losing fat they were gaining muscle, and the muscle they gained was not only heavier than the fat, it also took up much less body space.

When you first start the Lighten Up programme you may find that your weight will fluctuate a bit to begin with, especially if you've been yo-yo dieting. *Don't panic!* It takes the body a little while to readjust. Some people start to lose up to two pounds a week steadily right from Week One, while others will be two or three weeks into the programme before they see a consistent loss. This is absolutely fine – it took you a long time to gain the weight, so give yourself time to lose it. The great thing is that you'll be losing it without dieting and making yourself miserable, you'll be feeling positive and you'll really be enjoying your food. And when you do start to see a steady drop of between half a pound and two pounds of fat per week you can be very pleased with yourself because you know that this time it's a *permanent* fat dump.

Off the scales

 This is the form we give out to everybody at the beginning of the eight-week course. The only part you *have* to fill in is the goal statement at the beginning and you can either do this in the space provided or copy it out into your Lighten Up Diary. Whether you do the weighing and measuring is up to you. The important thing is to write down the goal or goals.

My Goals

What is your personal goal for this course? If you find that you have more than one just jot down everything you can think of, what you want to achieve, how you want to feel and how you might change the way you do things.

....

....

....

....

Current measurements:

Chest: ....

Upper Arm: .... (non-dominant arm)

Waist: ....

Hips: ....

Upper Leg: .... (specify left or right)

Calf: .... (specify left or right)

Weight: ....

Some other measurements

At Lighten Up we believe in feedback. Somebody once said that trying to lose weight without using scales is like ten-pin bowling without being allowed to see the pins. You roll your ball down the track but, at the moment of impact, a screen comes down and you've no idea what you scored.

Well, they have a point, but scales aren't the only way to measure how you're getting on. Feedback is certainly important, it keeps you going, gives you a sense of achievement and stops you getting fed up. But there are other ways of getting feed back than relying on the scales.

Make a note to ask yourself at the end of the second week and each week thereafter whether the following statements are true for you. These are the clues which will tell you that you're losing weight.

★ My clothes feel looser.
★ I have more energy.
★ I'm more active.
★ I'm looking forward to the Challenges at the end of each chapter.
★ I'm keeping my Lighten Up Diary and noticing patterns in my life that will give me the vital clues to change (more about this later).

Weighing is a ritual for a lot of people and they do it in the same way they eat, without thinking or asking themselves if it's what they want. We got by for thousands of years without scales and there are more life-giving things you could be doing with those few minutes every day. Like making up an Affirmation for yourself, or watering your plants or planning some non-food treats to take you through to bedtime.

BE YOUR OWN ROLE MODEL

Although we studied the habits and patterns of a lot of successful slimmers and naturally slim people when we were putting the Lighten Up programme together, Lighten Up isn't about living by somebody else's rules. One of the things we're going to keep repeating over the next eight weeks is that we want you to learn to trust yourself, to make your own decisions and to become your own role model.

Think of something positive you've done in your life. Something that meant cutting yourself off from other possibilities. Something you made a decision to do and then went ahead and did. And even though there might have been some setbacks, you carried on regardless because you knew, deep down, that you were going to achieve your goal.

It doesn't matter whether it turned out to be right or wrong. It's the process that matters.

I bought a car
I moved to a place of my own
I changed jobs
I went to college
I passed my exams
I gave up work to look after the kids
I learned to dance
I got married
I became independent
I adopted a cat
I started a business
I saved up for a holiday
I escaped . . .

Once you've chosen a memory or two, run a movie of those memories in your mind. Enjoy them for a few seconds and then, keeping the memories with you, make a firm commitment to yourself to be slimmer. Leave yourself no other option. True commitment to a decision always unlocks the energy to achieve it.

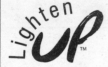 *Take at least ten minutes over this exercise and make a note about how it makes you feel in your Lighten Up Diary.*

THE POWER OF DECISIONS

What precedes all behaviours, actions and performances?

What turns dreams into reality?

The answer is *decisions*: *your decisions.* They determine what you think, how you feel, what you do and who you become.

Why are some people successful at becoming slimmer, fitter and healthier? Because they make better decisions. Because they make decisions full stop.

Most of us just hope, wish and, eventually, regret: 'I'm not good enough . . . I'm too old . . . I haven't had the right opportunities . . . I'm just a fat person . . .'

Successful slimmers give up hope and make a decision. How can you tell a decision from a hope, a wish – or even a fear? We've seen a lot of hopes and wishes and vague intentions cunningly disguised as decisions: decisions to take regular exercise, decisions to eat a healthy diet, decisions to change jobs . . . but these so-called decisions never lead anywhere. So how do you know when you've got the real thing, when you've made a real decision?

Real decisions trigger instant action. Hoping and wishing on the other hand are states of inactivity – almost paralysis.

When you think a thought and it changes everything, that thought was a decision.

We can give you the information you need to reach your goal, but the missing ingredient that only you can supply is the crucial decision that puts you on the road to change.

Of course, you are already taking action based on the last decision you made about your weight and it's producing the results you've got now. Eating to change the way you feel, constantly dieting and thinking about food, trying to stick to hard, damaging exercise routines are all actions which have produced results. But they probably weren't the results you wanted.

So why not make a *new* decision: one that will give you a happier, healthier lifestyle? The only discomfort you'll feel is a moment's anxiety about stepping outside your comfort zone.

Contract

 On the last page of your Lighten Up Diary write out the following statement, then sign and date it. This is your contract with yourself.

★ I'm willing to read this book and to honour my decision to become permanently slimmer and healthier.
★ I will write down what I eat and drink.

★ I will use the techniques and strategies in this book, and add to my life the ones that work for me.

★ I can and will achieve my personal goal (or goals). (Add in the words you wrote on page 108 when you wrote down your measurements. This is your goal statement, for now. Say it to yourself a hundred times a day, or more if you want.)

Signed .... Date ....

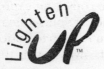 *Flip forward and look at this contract whenever you feel you need a bit of motivation.*

THE LIGHTEN UP DIARY

In Chapter Seven we talked about how you can increase the power and impact of your goals simply by writing them down. We've already invited you to write down your goal for the next eight weeks and suggested you sign a contract with yourself – but you're not through yet. We're finishing this week, as we will every week from now on, with the Diary.

And of course there's nothing revolutionary in that. Lots of diet books suggest you keep a diary. Some of them encourage you to write down every calorie you consume. But that's completely pointless unless you want to get even more obsessive about food than you are already.

And, yes, there are other diet books that ask you, as we do, to become more aware of your eating patterns. Well, that's because it's very useful to know more about when and where and why and how you eat. *What* you eat is less important at this stage, though we'll be asking you to record that as well – to begin with.

We are all creatures of habit and most of our daily routines are automatic. Writing things down can make you aware of personal behaviour patterns you never noticed before. And once you've noticed a bad habit you can start to change it. If you want to.

You can't tackle a problem you aren't even aware of.

HOW TO BE YOU

You've already started your notebook and the Diary is just a logical continuation of this. Put the date at the top of the page and write things down as they happen. It really doesn't matter how you do it, so long as you do it every day and take time to review your progress as the weeks go by.

It might help, as you're filling in your Diary, if you imagine that we've asked you to write a detailed daily instruction manual on how to be you. After a few weeks, anyone who reads that Diary should have enough detail to be able to copy your eating habits pretty accurately. What you find out about yourself may surprise you, even after just a few days, and you'll begin to notice more about what you do and when you do it. Awareness is the first step on the journey of change.

In the first few weeks the purpose of the Diary is to show you your eating and exercise patterns, so you can see what works and what doesn't. As the weeks go by you'll be adding in some other useful information about how you feel, what you drink and how much exercise you take and, after eight weeks, you'll know a lot about you. You need to have this information to make the changes that will make you slim and keep you slim.

But for the first week, all you need to do is make a note of:

★ *What* you eat and drink
★ *When* you eat and drink
★ *Activity* – walking, exercising, gardening – anything more than general pottering about
★ *Patterns* in your eating and drinking

For example . . .

Time	Food and Drinks	Activity
6 a.m.	Small packet Wotsits, Diet Coke	Walking to bus (15 minutes)
10 a.m.	Bacon sandwich, orange juice, coffee	Working

continued

Time	Food and Drinks	Activity
12.30 p.m.	Kebab and chips, mineral water	Working
5 p.m.	Banana, 2 cups tea	Working
6 p.m.	Mars bar	Walking home from the bus (15 minutes)
7 p.m.	2 cups tea	Watching TV
11 p.m.	Curry, rice, 2 pappadoms, 2 lagers, coffee	None

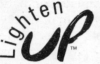

Fill in the Lighten Up Diary every day, several times a day to start with. At the beginning of the next seven chapters you will find a Diary review which will ask you to examine and compare your behaviour patterns and the changes you make to them week by week. Keep it simple but make it comprehensive. Write down everything at the time you eat it, don't wait until the end of the day. Don't judge or criticise or comment. Just notice your eating and exercise patterns and the other things you do around food.

CHALLENGES

At the end of each chapter, you'll find your Challenges for the week. These aim to help you move out of your comfort zone and start to change. For the first week they are quite simple and straightforward.

★ Get Moving: break the sedentary habit and start taking short, brisk exercise breaks whenever you find yourself sitting down for more than half an hour (some people even put the timer on their watch for this when they're watching TV).

★ Mind Your Language: run through your shoulds and oughts, and practise replacing them with cans and want tos every morning this week. You can do this while you clean your teeth, drink your morning cup of coffee, sit on the bus to work or whenever you have space to fit it in.

★ Think Thin: when you've practised the Open Door exercise with the book in front of you a couple of times, you'll be able to do it before you go to sleep at night and when you wake up in the morning.

★ Measure Your Success: measure yourself (weigh yourself if you have to!) and write down your chief goal for the programme. Then throw away the scales or donate them to a jumble sale.

★ Be Your Own Role Model: think of something you achieved that took the same kind of commitment and determination you're going to need for losing weight. Bear it in mind every time something in the programme seems a bit challenging. Whenever you think you'd like to weigh yourself (for example) stop and think of something you did well. It will help you resist the temptation to start rummaging through the dustbin for your scales.

★ The Power of Decisions: take control of your own life by making a decision to be slimmer and signing the contract.

★ And, most important, start your Lighten Up Diary today. It will be your personal support system for the next eight weeks.

Once you've got your head around the idea of being slimmer, fitter and healthier, your body will follow. And the Lighten Up programme is going to give you all the guidance and tools you need to get started.

Good Luck.

THE LIGHTEN UP CHECKLIST

Why do you need a Diary, a list of Challenges and a Checklist as well?

The Daily Checklist is just a practical little reminder to help you keep track of the core Lighten Up exercises for each week. The Diary and Challenges are different. They are flexible tools for change. After all, what you write in your Diary will depend on what's important to you and although for some people it's just a series of (very useful) lists, for others it will be a real, personal revelation. The Challenges are different again, usually one-offs or little practical things that you can do but not routines that have to be ticked off every day.

If you like, you could divide each day into sections and decide when you are going to do the exercises. For example, you might like to do the Mind Your Language exercise every day first thing in the morning and the Open Door visualisation at night. Everybody is different and your timing depends on you. So, all you have to do is make a decision and do it!

CHECKLIST FOR WEEK ONE

Daily checklist	*Day 1*	*Day 2*	*Day 3*	*Day 4*	*Day 5*	*Day 6*	*Day 7*
How many times did you get up and take a brisk walk around today?	☐	☐	☐	☐	☐	☐	☐
Mind Your Language exercise	☐	☐	☐	☐	☐	☐	☐
Open Door Visualisation	☐	☐	☐	☐	☐	☐	☐
The Lighten Up Diary	☐	☐	☐	☐	☐	☐	☐

WEEK TWO
OF THE
EIGHT-WEEK
COURSE

HOW ARE YOU DOING?

Some of you are probably wondering, 'Am I getting this right or wrong? This isn't like anything I've done before. I don't know whether I've lost any weight.' Not surprisingly, because some of you will have had experiences with past diets that have made you pessimistic.

The Lighten Up programme may be depriving you of your familiar dieting and weighing routines, but do you really want to go through all that again? If you haven't succeeded in losing weight permanently before, you definitely need to do things differently. You will soon start to see and feel positive changes that will reassure you that you're on the right track.

You'll soon find yourself developing a clearer picture of your habits as you become more aware of eating and of being more active every day. With this picture in front of you, it's much easier to see what progress you're making and what you still want to change.

LAST WEEK'S LIGHTEN UP DIARY AND CHALLENGES

At the beginning of every week we'll be reviewing how you got on with the programme during the previous week, starting with your Challenges and then taking a look back at what you wrote in the Lighten Up Diary. You won't need to keep referring back to the last chapter when you're going through this review – there should be enough here to remind you of what you were doing. But if you really feel you haven't done justice to all the ideas in the previous week the best thing is just to go right back to the beginning of it and do it again. After all, what's another week in a lifetime of change?

★ Did you get up and walk about regularly whenever you spent long periods in front of a screen or a desk? Have you noticed how active (or inactive) you are?

★ What have you learned from the Mind Your Language exercise? Will you find it easier to say things more positively in future?

★ How easy did you find the Open Door exercise? By now you can probably call up that picture of the Future You quite quickly.

★ Have you remembered some past successes and filed them away in your mind (or written them down in your Diary) ready to access whenever you need inspiration?

★ Look at the goal you wrote down. How do you feel about it now?

★ Are you honouring your decision to change?

★ Now let's look back over your Diary.

Take a look at the Diary you started last week. How easy was it for you to keep a daily record of what you were eating and drinking? What sort of patterns, habits or trends did you notice? Anything on the following list? Write the answers to these questions in your Diary, and go into detail. Really *think* about it. This exercise usually takes around 15 to 20 minutes and, if it takes longer, that's fine.

★ Are there any patterns to when and what you eat and drink?
★ Were there any surprises about how much (or how little) you eat and drink?
★ Are there particular times when you eat particular things?
★ Do you eat more at certain times of the day?
★ Where do you eat your meals (and snacks)?
★ Do you eat when you're bored?
★ Do you enjoy every bite?
★ How fast or slowly do you eat? Compared with friends? Compared with family?
★ Do you eat the same food as the people you share your meals with?
★ Do you eat differently when you're alone? More? Or less? Different kinds of food?
★ What is your favourite meal? Is it good for you?
★ Do you graze, or do you stick to three meals a day?
★ How far ahead of time do you plan what you're going to eat?
★ Do you enjoy your food as much as you did ten years ago? More? Or less?
★ Do you eat as much as you did ten years ago? More? Or less?
★ Does your favourite food make you happy? While you're eating it? Afterwards?
★ Is there something you can't resist?
★ Do you have any activities that trigger you to eat?
★ Can you imagine living without your favourite food for six weeks?
★ Which meal have you enjoyed the most in the last seven days? What was good about it?
★ How much time do you spend thinking about food?
★ How much time do you spend preparing food?
★ What food feels best in your stomach after you've eaten it?
★ What food smells best before you eat it?

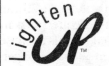

Write a short summary of the last week for yourself. What did you notice most? What really stood out?

Are You Ready?

It is always advisable to check with your doctor before starting on this or any other diet and fitness programme. Most people will benefit from taking exercise, but do consult with your doctor if you feel that there may be some doubt as to your suitability.

 WEEK TWO

This week, as well as tackling some new concepts like the Fat Jar and the Hunger Scale, you'll also be working on more advanced versions of ideas you were introduced to last week, such as visualisation and making positive statements. The more you practise these, the more benefit you'll get from them. Below is a summary of what we're going to be focusing on this week. Find yourself a place where you won't be disturbed and take the time to work through this chapter, trying out the ideas and acting on the 'Do This Now' exercises. At the end, you'll find your Challenges for the week, together with your daily checklist.

★ The Exercise Wheel: being more active is very important if you want to be slim.
★ The Fat Jar: leading a more active life.
★ Calories Are Wasted if They're Not Tasted: taking the time to enjoy your food instead of hurrying it and worrying about it.
★ Common Eating Patterns: becoming more aware of why and when you eat.
★ The Hunger Scale: learning to eat because you're hungry.
★ A Healthy Diet: it's time to start thinking about what you eat as well as how and when and why.
★ Slimming From the Head Down: practising positive visualisation and introducing goal setting and affirmations.

THE EXERCISE WHEEL

What you do – or rather, how much you do – is very important if you want to be slim. And no, this isn't about going to the gym, so even if you loathe exercise, keep reading. At this stage in the Lighten Up programme we just want you to think about being a little more active in your daily life. In fact, even if you do decide later on to do some regular exercise, the real key to losing weight is to adjust your daily routine so that you become less sedentary.[1]

A few weeks ago I volunteered to help a friend of mine organise the games for her little boy's birthday party. I haven't been in a confined space with so many five-year-olds since I was at school myself, and after an hour I was exhausted. The energy levels at that party were higher than the aerobic classes I used to lead! I'd forgotten how children run around all the time. They're constantly in motion. Which is why you don't see as many overweight children as overweight adults. (Though there are more of them now than there used to be because they don't seem to walk to school and play out in the street any more – I suppose they're stuck indoors with their Playstations.)

Our bodies are designed to do one thing and one thing only: move. The main fuel that powers them is fat. And, if we don't use our bodies today, the fuel gets stored for tomorrow.

We drive to work. We're just as likely to take the lift to the second floor as to the twenty-second. We sit down in front of a screen all day, then we go home and sit down in front of a screen all evening, pausing only to order a pizza when we think we ought to be hungry. Fitting in the average 26 hours a week television viewing doesn't leave much time for dancing, cooking or even taking the kids out to play games. And yet we complain about feeling tired all the time.

The environment we live in does nothing to encourage activity. We don't have to work the land or chase our food – we can even order groceries over the Internet and have them delivered if we really don't want to run the risk of depleting any of our fat cells before stocking up again.

1 'These folks have found the secret of being able to incorporate exercise into their lives,' Dr Jim Hill, Co-Director of the US National Weight Loss Registry, describing a study of the 5 per cent of people who maintained a 30lb weight loss for more than a year.

So we don't get much exercise out of necessity and most of us don't go out and exercise for fun either. PE at school cured us of that, and the associations of discomfort, humiliation and goosebumps linger on. And, not surprisingly, slogans like 'No Pain No Gain' and 'Go for the Burn' have only reinforced the general aversion. So how do we at Lighten Up go about convincing people who think they dislike exercise that it can be comfortable and fun?

The answer (as usual) is *pleasure* – it's what motivates us all. Out there, somewhere, is a fun form of exercise for everybody. Do something you enjoy and which gives you pleasure, whether this is a walk in the park, a round of golf or a dance class. What you do doesn't matter – what's important is that you're doing something. Enjoyable, comfortable activity is the best way to break up fat cells. You don't need a punishing gym routine. You can be active enough to burn fat without ever moving out of your comfort zone – active people have more trained muscle, which burns fat to maintain itself even when they're just sitting watching television.

Exercise patterns

Examples of exercise patterns, already filled in:

Typical working day	Typical relaxing day
6 hours sleep	8 hours sleep
11 hours sitting	7 hours sitting
4 hours pottering	7 hours pottering
1 hour walking etc. (Fat Jar Fitness)	1 hour walking etc. (Fat Jar Fitness)
2 hours travelling	1 hour exercise (Feelgood Fitness)

Each segment in the examples opposite is an hour of the day. Photocopy an empty wheel for every day of the week and fill it in as you keep your Diary, using different colours or shading for each of the six categories shown in the key.

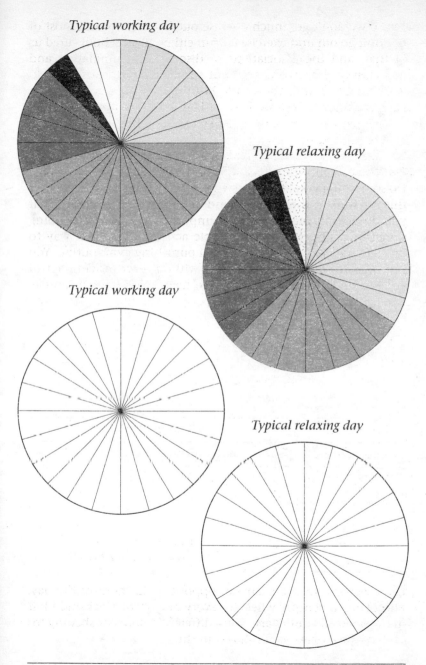

Typical working day

Typical relaxing day

Typical working day

Typical relaxing day

Key

Sleeping.

Sitting: working at a desk or VDU, eating, watching TV, travelling.

Pottering about: light housework, office work, shopping.

Fat Jar Fitness: walking/cycling/stairs/escalators: going somewhere fast without breaking a sweat.

Travelling: driving or public transport.

Feel Good Fitness: sport, aerobics, circuit training, running, dancing, weight training (more details about this in Week Three).

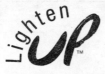

Over the next few weeks, see if you can include more activity in your life and even out the balance between the two wheels.

The five per cent solution

Once you start filling in your Exercise Wheel regularly, you'll get a clearer idea of whether you're getting enough exercise. You simply weren't designed to spend your life sitting down!

Remember the 5 per cent of people who manage to lose weight and keep it off? I can assure you that the exercise that does the trick for them isn't daily aerobics or marathon running. It's walking and cycling and gardening and cleaning and playing football with children – the kind of thing we all used to do more often and could probably do again. At Lighten Up we call it Fat Jar Fitness and we'll be explaining more about that later

There are lots of everyday activities that count as good exercise. And, when you're ready, you can add in some extra ones that turn up your metabolic thermostat, but which don't have to involve complicated arrangements at the gym or the squash court – unless you want them to.

How many of these do you already do and how many could you add?

Activity	Already do it?	Times per week?	Add it?
Walking to work	_____	_____	_____
Walking part of the way to work	_____	_____	_____
Walking to the shops/school	_____	_____	_____
Recreation involving exercise	_____	_____	_____
Cycling instead of other transport	_____	_____	_____
Walking up stairs and escalators	_____	_____	_____
Running up stairs	_____	_____	_____
Getting up hourly at work and stretching	_____	_____	_____
Mini-stretch programme while watching TV	_____	_____	_____
Housework	_____	_____	_____
Gardening	_____	_____	_____
Outdoor games with children	_____	_____	_____
Walking a dog	_____	_____	_____
What else?	_____	_____	_____

How easy will it be to add more activity into your routine?

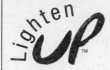

This week, add in one of these suggested activities every day – you'll find a space for it on the daily checklist at the end of the chapter.

Take it easy

Being overweight is a vicious circle because our body chemistry favours stability. Overweight people tend to take less exercise than thin ones because it's harder for them – they don't build as much muscle as thin people do and it's muscle that burns fat. So when muscle gives way to fat through inactivity, they burn less of that fat when they *do* exercise.

It takes far more calories to maintain a pound of muscle in your body than to maintain a pound of fat. Even when muscles are inactive, they burn more calories than fat does.

The Lighten Up programme encourages you to be more active but we do take on board how difficult this might be for some people and it's understandable that a lot of overweight people prefer to diet rather than exercise. Unfortunately, the sad truth is that dieting slows down the metabolism and, after dieting for two weeks, your metabolic rate can drop by 20 per cent. So being fat makes you even fatter (because fat people don't have enough muscle to burn the calories) and dieting makes it worse by slowing down your metabolism.

Fat people get exhausted and breathless when they exercise too hard because their bodies are trying to maintain the status quo by saving fat and burning sugar (glucose). The outcome is painful, disheartening and doesn't result in fat reduction. That's why I'm telling you to take it very gently at first. Forget the sweat and the lycra, and just do as much exercise as you enjoy.

As you become more active, your shape will begin to change, you'll feel healthier – and you might start to wonder how you managed without those good feelings you get from gentle, steady, regular exercise.

All you need now is your Fat Jar.

THE FAT JAR

Be a fat-burning machine, not a fat-storing machine.

Fifteen minutes of continuous activity seems to be the time trigger necessary to stimulate the production of fat-burning enzymes. The more enzymes you have, the more fat you can burn. But although it takes fifteen minutes to produce new enzymes, you ones you already have will be burning fat from the very first step you take.

 Get yourself a jar. Every time you walk briskly for fifteen minutes, put a five-pence piece into it. If you're at work, or out for the day simply make a note of it and put the coins into your Fat Jar later. That way you can *see* how active you are and how much more active you are becoming. Every coin is a Lighten Up Fat-Burning Pill. They are safe and effective, and when your jar is full you can use them to buy yourself a non-fattening treat. You'll have earned it.

A lot of diets suggest it's hard to burn fat but that's not actually true. We're burning fat all the time. Seventy per cent of our muscles' energy needs come from fat and the main point of exercise is to work those muscles just that bit harder and longer so as to burn more of it.

Burning calories is another benefit, but this tends to get overemphasised because we forget that we're burning calories all the time, even when we're asleep. You might only burn a couple of biscuits' worth in an exercise session but that doesn't matter, don't think about it like that. Counting the calories you burn is as depressing and obsessive as counting the calories you eat. Forget about it. Calorie burning is the least important part of exercise. The main reason for being more active is to become more efficient at using fat as your major energy source instead of storing it.

The more exercise you do, the more your metabolism will speed up. Not only will you digest food more quickly, you'll also be building lean muscle, which uses more calories than fat. But this takes time – if you want to change something as fundamental as your body chemistry, you have to do it at a pace which suits your body. That might mean telling your mind to be patient. While you're waiting it helps to remember that every time you walk up the escalator or leave the car in the garage, you are turning up your internal thermostat and burning more fuel.

The main criterion for exercise is that it should be comfortable and continuous.

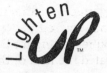 Get yourself a Fat Jar and aim to put in at least five pence a day for this week.

CALORIES ARE WASTED
IF THEY'RE NOT TASTED

Well, so much for exercise, this week at least. Let's get on to the eating habits that may be slowing down the slimming process for you.

When I first met Mo, one of the original Lighten Uppers, I could guarantee that if I visited her while she was watching *East-Enders* I'd find her eating a big bag of Kettle Chips. When I teased her about this and tried to steal some she'd just snatch the packet away saying, 'Leave me alone, it's my half-hour of guaranteed pleasure at the end of a hard day.' They made her feel good. Until I messed things up by encouraging her to start tasting every mouthful.

She noticed that the first two or three handfuls tasted pretty good. Then there were eight or nine handfuls in between which she paid little attention to. The last few handfuls were good again because she realised her treat was almost over. And as she tossed the bag into the bin she'd feel dissatisfied, fat or full. She'd ask herself why she'd eaten all those crisps in the first place.

Eventually she decided that the eight or nine handfuls in the middle of the bag were unnecessary calories and stopped eating after the first two or three handfuls she enjoyed. (She discovered that if you fold over the top of the bag and clip it with a clothes peg, they still taste OK the next day.)

Although I haven't mentioned the word yet this week, what we're really talking about here are *habits*. And if you read Chapter Five, you'll know that getting to grips with your habits is an important part of the Lighten Up programme.

We all have eating and exercise habits that aren't necessarily good for us and perhaps don't even give us that much pleasure any more. But they've been around for a long time. Whether it's popcorn at the pictures (regardless of whether you're having a pizza afterwards) or a Crunchie bar while you're waiting for the train after work, your own brain once generated the idea of the habit because it thought it would make you happy. And now, here you are, stuck with it.

So when you're tired after a hard day, or someone upsets you, or you feel lonely, and your brain suggests food, don't punish yourself about it. Just noticing this behaviour is already helping you get slimmer. If you want to keep this habit you can, but if you don't, *you now have a choice.*

COMMON EATING PATTERNS

Many things we do are automatic. And that's the way they ought to be. If a centipede stopped to work out which leg to move next, it would never get started again. Breathing is just one of many functions that our subconscious manages very well without our conscious involvement and digestion is another. But there are some activities we hand over to our subconscious which we should perhaps become more aware of and monitor more closely.

| DO THIS NOW | Do you recognise any of these? Tick any habits that look familiar. |

Skipping breakfast ☐

Skipping breakfast and then having a doughnut and coffee mid-morning ☐

Eating on the go ☐

Eating in the car ☐

Eating to stay awake at the computer ☐

Eating too much of one or two particular types of food ☐

Eating something sugary late afternoon ☐

Eating just to soak up the beer ☐

Ordering takeaways when you're too tired to cook ☐

Skipping meals altogether ☐

Substituting sweet or fatty snacks for meals ☐

Eating while watching TV ☐

Deciding it's easier to grab a biscuit than peel an orange ☐

Eating the biggest meal of the day late in the evening when your most strenuous activity will be picking up the remote control ☐

Eating when you're bored, angry, sad, happy or excited ☐

Eating for any reason other than hunger ☐

Did your Diary for the past week reveal any other patterns that you have? List them here:

....

If you do any of the above, and think they might be contributing to your weight problem, could you change them?

Decide on five eating patterns you'd like to do without and put them in order of importance. Start a new page in your Diary and head it 'Eating Patterns'. Then write down the five patterns you don't like. Read them through a couple of times and make a personal commitment to getting rid of them. Do one at a time if you don't think you can eliminate them all at once. Start with the one at the top of the list and make it your target for this week.

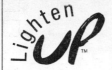

If you don't recognise any of the patterns on the list, see if you can think of any other eating habits you have that you could do without and tackle those instead.

THE HUNGER SCALE

At last, some scales!

The Hunger Scale is one you can use for the rest of your life; it's accurate, reliable and you can even take it on holiday with you.

Eating when we're not physically hungry is the second most common cause of being overweight. (The first is not taking enough exercise.) If we eat when we aren't hungry, our bodies just store the food we don't need as fat. Once we stop eating when we aren't hungry, control is back in our hands.

The Hunger Scale is an incredibly effective way of doing this. Once you start using it regularly you'll find you get better at ignoring your normal eating triggers and you'll learn to recognise a new one – hunger. Your relationship with food will improve as you begin to notice whether or not you're hungry.

Whenever you think it might be lunchtime or you fancy a sandwich, stop and ask yourself first, 'How hungry am I on a scale of one to ten?'

 next time you eat: Record the date, time and Hunger Scale figure in your Lighten Up Diary.

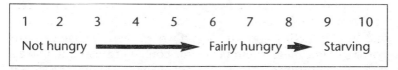

If you register 6 or above, you're probably quite hungry. If you register 5 or below, you probably aren't; 6, 7 and 8 on the scale are showing true physical hunger. If you get to 9 or 10 you're really starving and probably haven't eaten for some time. If you let yourself get to this point you will be in danger of overeating once you start. (And don't worry, there are more details about how to gauge your hunger accurately coming up on the next page.)

Many people are afraid to eat for pleasure and they've forgotten how to eat when they're hungry. Most diets tell you to ignore hunger and abstain from pleasure, and they also tell you when, how much and exactly what to eat. No wonder we've lost touch with our bodies' natural responses to our physical and emotional needs.

The subliminal message on the cover of any diet book is this: *Human beings are unable to manage their bodies and eating patterns.* But it's simply not true. In fact, the reverse is true. It's *not* listening to what our bodies are telling us that makes us overweight. But people go along with the diet myth because they think it will be easier than exercising and they love the security of being on a diet. It's also much easier to blame a diet for being too difficult to stick to or not giving results than it is to admit you've failed again.

Our goal is to teach you how to listen to yourself and your body, and to relearn what's right for you instead of living by a set of somebody else's rules.

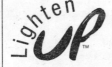 Don't worry if you don't think you can do this at the moment, just pretend you can for the rest of the week and see how you feel about it by the end.

Am I hungry?

So what techniques can you use to judge where you are on the Hunger Scale? How easily can you tell the difference between hunger and tension, or hunger and boredom?

SOME SIGNS OF HUNGER

★ Smelling or tasting a food you want when it's not there
★ Knowing exactly what you want to eat
★ Empty feelings in the stomach
★ Sharp, but not unpleasant sensations in the stomach, accompanied by rumbling
★ Loss of energy
★ Irritability
★ Light-headedness
★ Slightly nauseous headache accompanied by desire to eat
★ Sudden fall in motivation for the task in hand
★ Inability to think about anything but food

 Check to see if you have any signs of hunger. If you're not sure whether you're hungry or not, you're probably not.

If I'm not hungry, what am I?

Everybody's different, and what we want is for you really to get to know yourself. So before you assume that your rumbling stomach or nauseous headache means hunger – **stop!** Run a few internal tests to help you to get to know what hungry means for you. Are you:

★ Bored with what you're doing and looking for something to distract you?
★ Tired? (eating can wake you up and give you an energy boost, but it might be better just to take a nap – or go for a walk).
★ Tense or anxious? (have you noticed your stomach tends to rumble or contract in interviews).
★ Thirsty? (easily confused with hunger, especially if the craving's for something juicy).
★ Clock watching? (so what if it's teatime).
★ Angry? (a cup of tea and a chocolate digestive have a calming effect).
★ Lonely? (eating's the next best thing to having company).

- ★ Depressed? (there's nothing like a piece of fudge cake to cheer you up).
- ★ In need of comfort? (some days – and some parts of the day – can seem pretty bleak).
- ★ Needing to chew or suck something? (this is a fairly primitive one).
- ★ Remembering good times past? (this happens sometimes when you see appetising food and recall eating and enjoying something similar).
- ★ Suffering from indigestion? (can be confused with hunger pangs).

Remember that the cliché 'hungry for love' is overused, but for a very good reason: we often try to satisfy emotional needs with food – it's sometimes easier to fill the gap in your life by ordering a takeaway than it is to tackle the root of the problem.

Even if you're convinced you really are hungry, before you go ahead and eat . . .

DOUBLE CHECK!

- ★ If you have food in front of you, smell it before tasting it. If it doesn't smell perfect, don't eat it.
- ★ Ask yourself, 'Would anything other than food satisfy me right now?'

COPING WITH CRAVINGS

If you're hit by a craving that's hard to resist, but deep down you know that it's nothing to do with hunger, this is what you do:

- ★ Never give in to it immediately, cravings always come in waves and it will subside.
- ★ Make it easier for yourself by doing something else until the craving has passed. Anything that involves moving away from the fridge is a good idea, so taking a short walk or making a phone call often work well. We'll be giving you lots more ideas for displacement activities later in the programme.

A HEALTHY DIET

It's finally time to start thinking about *what* you eat as well as how and when and why.

The foods we eat are made up of:

★ carbohydrates
★ fats
★ proteins
★ vitamins and minerals
★ water

When we ask people at Lighten Up workshops to describe their idea of a healthy diet most of the instant answers include the word 'varied'. So why do we continue to fall for the milkshake or grapefruit-and-steak diets? And why do we eat monotonously fatty foods instead of taking the trouble to prepare fruit and vegetables? The majority of people seem to know quite a lot about healthy diets in theory, but they don't take their own advice.

Our bodies need nutrients from all the food groups if we are to function properly. Dietary advice has changed many times over the past thirty years and some of the information can occasionally appear to conflict, but don't give up. The key is to eat a wide variety of all types of fresh foods rather than cutting out one or more of the food groups completely. And at the back of this book, in Section Three, we've included the most up-to-date information on health and nutrition for you to refer to and dip into whenever you feel you want to know more.

There is no magic diet that guarantees weight loss.

So forget the pineapple diet and aim for balance rather than perfection. Eat what you enjoy. Of course, this doesn't mean you should eat chocolate eclairs three times a day, but one cream slice once in a while isn't so terrible and certainly nothing to be ashamed of or hate yourself for.

There is no 'perfect' diet either.

Our bodies and preferences are all different and there's no set of rules which could guarantee the perfect diet for everyone. Go for variety and balance, and make sure you eat things you can enjoy – especially those which aren't too sweet or deep-fried.

Above all, remember that natural, fresh products are best because the human body has had years and years of practice at digesting them and can convert them easily into energy. Foods that are pre-prepared and packaged are more likely to be chemically enhanced or preserved and our gut has only had a few years to get used to these new substances. They confuse our bodies and are difficult to digest.

You are what you eat

 No need to write these answers in the Diary. Just go through them in your head.

★ Do you think you have a balanced diet?
★ Does it include plenty of fresh fruit and vegetables?
★ How, specifically, do the foods you eat make you feel?
★ How do you prepare your food?
★ What foods are you drawn towards and feel compelled to eat? Are they good for you?
★ Do you know why you like some things and not others? (Unmashed tinned tomatoes in school dinners or eating a dodgy prawn can put you off some perfectly nutritious foods for life.)
★ Are there any foods you like the look of but have never tasted?
★ Are there some foods you've never eaten but *know* you wouldn't like?
★ Do you eat certain types of food at certain times of day? Do you know why this is?
★ Can you smell some foods when they aren't around? Cucumber? Garlic? Melted cheese? Chips with vinegar? Chocolate? Bread? If you divided the foods you can smell without seeing them into separate lists, which would be the longest? Would it be fruit and vegetables? Sweet things? Salty, savoury food?

Over the next few weeks you'll become more aware of your patterns and associations with food, and you're going to start changing some of them for ever.

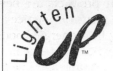

Come back to the list and read it again before starting to write your Lighten Up Diary for this week.

SLIMMING FROM THE HEAD DOWN

If you think we are going round in circles, bear with us and keep practising. We're going to keep on doing this until it's part of you and you can throw away the book and get on with your life.

Most people have a tendency to focus on what's not working, that's to say, they obsess about problems. Which is a pity, really, because our brains work much more efficiently with positive commands. In fact, as we're about to prove, the human brain deletes negatives.

 If you say to yourself 'I must not *keep eating*,' guess what message you get?

Say to yourself, 'I must lose *weight*.' Write down what you see when you say it.

What happens when you say to yourself 'I am going to *be slimmer*'? What picture do you get this time? How is it different from the previous one?

In life you get what you focus on. All great achievers owe their success to their ability to focus on exactly what it is that they want. Haven't you met people like that? They'll be the ones going on and on about having a dream or a vision, while everybody else is complaining about working long hours for low pay. So if you get what you focus on, what, exactly, have you been focusing on so far?

Your brain will home in on whatever is put in front of it. The trick is to tell yourself what you want, *not* what you don't want. If you are watching your weight, that is *exactly* what you will keep seeing. Depressing, isn't it?

Start putting your aims and goals and dreams for a slimmer future into positive terms. An architect has to draw up detailed plans before starting to build a house and your vision of how *you* want to be needs to be as detailed as the architect's drawings.

 Open up your Lighten Up Diary to a new page and write or draw a clear description of the new you. You can refer to it whenever the picture grows dim or you need a flash of inspiration. As you look at what you've jotted down, an image may appear in your mind. Perhaps it's already sharply defined, in bright, clear colours. Or maybe it's slowly taking shape. Give it the attention it deserves.

Every great achievement flashes through the mind before it turns into reality. But you don't have to wait for flashes of inspiration; you can use your imagination to create your own.

A wide-screen technicolour expert

Most people see themselves as they think they are. *If you want to be successful, see yourself as you would like to be.*

Everybody daydreams. Some people are better at it than others but whether it comes naturally or not, you can become a wide-screen, technicolour expert if you concentrate and work harder at your daydreaming technique.

What makes great artists better than the rest? Their ability to visualise the result they want to achieve. Once they have a clear and vividly imagined picture in their minds, they are more than halfway to achieving it.

And what about some of the greatest inventors and innovators? Take Einstein. When he came up with $E = mc^2$ he wasn't poring over equations in black and white. He was imagining what it would be like to travel on a light beam! In fact, Einstein, one of the greatest scientists in history, always maintained that imagination was more important than knowledge. Our imaginations are grossly neglected, considering how extremely useful they can be as tools for change. Most of us only use them for recreational purposes – or for upsetting ourselves if we happen to be worriers.

A lot of this probably goes back to childhood. When you were at school, gazing out of the window, imagining yourself on wild adventures, the teachers probably told you to stop wasting time and pay attention. Daydreaming was discouraged and imagination was a waste of time. Yet if you speak to successful people (who often didn't do too well at conventional education) they will tell you that they used to dream. Steven Spielberg was always convinced that he was going to make not just regular movies, but blockbusters, because he'd done it in his imagination so many times.

A lot of people think they can't visualise, but we all think in pictures. If somebody asks you 'What did you have for dinner last night?' or 'Tell me about your holiday', you'll be seeing it in your mind before you start putting it into words .

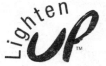 Psychologists believe that in order to really fix something in your mind, you need to repeat it twenty times. You can do the following exercise twenty times if you like (not all at once), but there's nothing to stop you doing it thirty or forty. The more you practise, the more likely you are to get what you want.

WHAT DO YOU WANT?

 You've already stretched your mind a bit. So stretch it a little more while you're feeling flexible. Ask yourself these questions. You don't have to write down the answers in your Diary (we've given you some examples) but it helps.

What do you want? Be very specific about it.
I want to be as slim as I was before I got married.

When do you want it?
By the time I go on holiday, five months from now.

Where do you want it?
I want to look slimmer all over – the tops of my arms, my face, my thighs and, of course, my bum.

Whom do you want it with?
I know it matters to my partner. He doesn't nag me, but I caught him looking at some of our honeymoon photos the other day. I looked wonderful in those photos. And that was only ten years ago.

What would be different as a result of you achieving this?
I'd be able to go swimming with the children and wear short skirts again.

What would achieving this do for you?
It would do wonders for my self-esteem.

What would achieving this get for you?
Respect.

What would achieving this give you?
It would give me the confidence to join in with more social activities and start having fun again.

What resources do you have to accomplish this?
Having the children wasn't easy. I gave up smoking, I gave up work when I had my second one and I gave up some of my identity. But I knew that I wanted to be a mother so the sacrifices were worth it and I persevered. I have a lot of determination and also a lot of self-worth, which helped me survive.

What is it about you that will allow you to do it?
Knowing that I can be different, that I can be slim and attractive again. I have this conviction inside me that it is possible.

What additional resources do you need to achieve this?
I could do with some external support. I think that getting together with a couple of friends so that we can work through the ideas together will keep me going when I hit my usual 'give up the diet after three weeks' syndrome.

How will you know when you've achieved it?
I have a couple of swimsuits I haven't worn for years and a ballgown too. If I could wear them again, it would be just wonderful.

What will you be seeing, hearing feeling, smelling and tasting?
I'll be seeing an image I like in the mirror. I'll be hearing compliments – and bitchy comments, too! There's always somebody who hates it when you change. I know I'll be feeling more energetic – it would be nice to go upstairs without getting breathless. And I've started to think about the different foods I'll be eating, what they're going to smell and taste like. I'm concentrating on good smells like strawberries, and tasting salads with cucumber and fresh herbs.

What will you look like and sound like when you've achieved this?
I'm going to look glamorous and I'm going to sound sexy.

What will happen if you achieve this?
I plan to take salsa lessons on the night my partner looks after the children.

What won't happen if you achieve this?
I won't be staying at home watching TV as much as I do now.

What would you get to have or keep by *not* achieving this?
They way my life is now may not be exciting but it's comfortable. I don't have to make much effort about my appearance, for example – it's hardly worth it when I know that anything fashionable is going to emphasise how fat I am. And what's the point of make-up when nobody's looking at my face?

How do you know that your goal is worth achieving?
Because I can still remember what it was like to flirt, to feel attractive, and feel like I had the right to go out and have fun.

How will achieving this affect your life, your family, your business, your job and your friends?
It's going to affect my job – I've already had one warning about not getting promotion because my image is wrong. That was another factor in my decision; now that I'm working full time again, I want to get back on the career ladder. My partner is going to like the change, but some of the friends I've made since I had the children might find the new me quite hard to accept. I'm definitely in the 'fat and jolly'

category at the moment, and switching to the sexy and successful one might cause a bit of a stir.

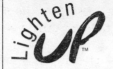 This exercise will be easier for some people than for others, but practice really will make perfect, so persevere.

Goal setting

Goal setting isn't something you do once and then get on with your life. Effective goal setting needs to become as much a part of your life as cleaning your teeth or paying your bills. It's an ongoing process and, at the end of every week from now on, after you've put the last tick in your check box on the last page of the chapter, we're going to suggest you review your slimming goal and write it out again. It doesn't matter whether it changes or not, week by week. Some weeks you may find it's evolved and some weeks it will be the same. If you got it right first time round it may stand just as you wrote it in the first week like a beacon for you to aim at. That's fine, but writing it down will still reinforce it for you and help you to stay focused.

WHAT DO YOU WANT?

Why are we asking you questions rather than telling you what to do?

Because Lighten Up is a process of change and in order to make changes you have to start questioning the way things are. Questioning what you want and where you're going, and giving yourself positive answers, is a good way to review your goals.

You've already practised making positive statements in Chapter One so what you just wrote may be wonderfully positive – in which case just carry on focusing on that positive goal.

But the negative habits of a lifetime die hard. If the first thing that flashes into your mind when you're faced with the 'What Do You Want' question is something like this:

I must stop eating so much
I want to cut out fat and sugar
I don't want to wear these baggy clothes any more

you may find your mind filling up with images of constant snacks, slabs of fat, bags of sugar and rails and rails of clothes you don't want to wear.

If you find that thoughts like these are still creeping in, stop and think. Then have another go. This time, when you hear the words 'What Do You Want?' think of something that fills your mind with pictures of you looking slim, healthy, happy, glowing and vital.

I want to be fitter, slimmer and healthier.
I want to look great in a swimsuit.
I want to buy fashionable clothes.
I want to get admiring glances when I walk into a room.
I want to feel good about myself.

This may sound repetitive, but for the next seven weeks we want you to keep checking the level of positivity in the way you talk to yourself. Eventually this will become automatic, but just keep an eye on the situation for the time being.

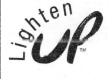 *As the weeks go by, you will get used to asking yourself, 'What Do I Want?' You will also get used to the fact that the answers tend to change as you do. That's fine, as long as your answer's always a positive one.*

Affirmations

What's the difference between an affirmation and a goal? An affirmation tells you that your goal is happening; it's an action statement about what's taking place *right now*. It inspires you and reassures you.

If your goal is 'I want to be slim' or 'I expect to be slim', your affirmation will be 'I'm getting slimmer every day'.

An affirmation is simply a motivational tool, like a compass, that you can use all day, every day to keep yourself moving in the right direction.

And, yes, it is a cliché, like 'thinking thin'. But it works, so it's worth doing. In fact, affirmations are a bit like goal setting – people know about them but are too embarrassed to use them. But what's more embarrassing – being publicly overweight and out of control, or privately giving yourself some encouragement?

Make up an affirmation

It should be a phrase that instantly conjures up a picture of yourself, looking and feeling the way you want to be.

For example:

I'm slim and getting slimmer.
I'm fit and getting fitter.
I'm becoming more like the person I want to be every day.

 Choose an Affirmation and write it below. It may be slightly different from your goal – something that supports it, perhaps. Or it might be exactly the same as your goal, but turned into an Affirmation – as if it's actually happening rather than something you're aiming for in the future.

....

....

★ When you repeat this Affirmation, try to picture yourself clearly being this way.

★ Make the image big, bright, bold and colourful; feel what it's like to have what you want.

★ Practise this over and over, repeating your Affirmation as many times as possible each day: you can do this in the shower, on the bus or while cooking your evening meal – any time you're doing something that leaves your mind free to focus on this. Repetition is the mother of all skill. If you tell yourself what you want over and over again (twenty times) and vividly imagine it, you will move closer and closer to your outcome.

★ Keep this mental picture (or movie) with you wherever you go.

 This is a good time to repeat the Open Door exercise. This time, when you step into the future you, repeat your Affirmation to yourself – with feeling.

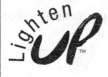 *All Affirmations sound silly at first (especially if you're British). Start quietly and build them up. Try really to believe in your Affirmation as you say it, but don't worry if you find it difficult at first.*

Think positive, speak positive

We haven't finished with being positive yet. In fact, you're never going to finish with it because you're going to be positive for life from now on. And it's not just a question of what you say. Weight loss starts in your mind. Think thin.

Many successful people say they owe their achievements to messages they constantly repeated to themselves over and over again: 'I will be famous, I will be rich . . .'

On the other hand, many unsuccessful people also owe their failures to the compelling messages they've been repeating to themselves: 'I'm fat . . . I'm useless . . . I'm just not lucky . . . My face doesn't fit . . .'

As I'm going to keep saying, you get what you focus on and your thoughts will expand to fit the available space. So, as Emerson and Gandhi both said, it's a good idea to think about what you want, rather than what you don't want.

We take the miracle of thought for granted. There are limitations to what you can do with your body (though not as many as you think) but your mind has no limits at all. Whatever you can dream of is waiting for you, so continue to spend your time constructively, thinking about being the way you want to be.

Lighten UP™

An ideal time to repeat your Affirmation is when you're taking your Fat-Burning Pills. You've got a head start because you're using your body anyway. The more often you repeat your Affirmation to yourself, the easier it will be to believe and the more quickly you will reach your goals.

THE LIGHTEN UP DIARY

New Notes

★ This week, as you write your Diary, take the time to photocopy or draw and fill in the Exercise Wheel as well. Notice how much of your time is spent not doing very much and see whether you can change this.

★ Were you doing anything else while you were eating?

★ Beside every entry, note what it was that triggered you to eat (time of day, opportunity for a break, someone else's invitation, hunger . . .).

★ Every time you eat, make a note of where you were on the Hunger Scale.

★ Notice, as you write, the range of food you eat. How varied – or how limited – is it?

★ How was the food prepared? Grilled? Poached? Raw? Sauces or dressings?

★ Start consciously looking for patterns as you become more aware of how, when and what you eat. You might find that you are changing some habits you never even knew you had.

Carry on

★ making a note of everything you eat and drink;

★ looking for *patterns* in your eating and drinking.

An Example (we'll discuss Triggers in Week Three):

WEEK 2

Time	Food and Drinks	Activity (and Trigger)	Hunger Scale (1–10)
7.30 a.m.	1 bowl unsweetened muesli, 1 coffee with semi-skimmed milk, orange juice	None	3
10.30 a.m.	Doughnut and black coffee	Read newspaper (always share coffee and snack when papers are delivered to office)	6
1.45 p.m.	Soup, wholemeal roll, apple, orange, banana, Diet Coke	Working	7
3 p.m.	Large Twix	New deadline to meet (needed calming down)	4
6.30 p.m.	2 cups of tea	Doing crossword (force of habit)	4
8.30 p.m.	Chicken and chips, salad, grapes, handful of nuts and raisins, 3 glasses of wine, ½ pint of water	None	6

CHALLENGES

★ Put at least one Fat-Burning Pill a day in the Fat Jar – that's 15 minutes of basic activity in addition to any activity you would normally do. But this isn't 'going to the gym' type of activity, it's normal stuff like extra walking or cycling, or not using the lift, or everyday jobs like gardening and house-work.

★ Use the Hunger Scale every time you eat.
★ Set aside five minutes night and morning to do some visual-isation of how you want to be.
★ Make up an Affirmation for yourself and say it night and morning.
★ Continue to keep the Lighten Up Diary and follow the sug-gestions on the previous page.
★ Review your goal when you come to the end of the week.

Note: Your goal may still be the same as the one you chose last week, but write it down again here. Sometimes you may not notice until you've actually written it down that your language has changed slightly – perhaps it sounds a bit more confident this time. But whether it's changed or not doesn't matter, just check that it's positive and inspiring, and keep it in mind until you make a new one.

CHECKLIST FOR WEEK TWO

Weekly checklist

Which eating pattern are you going to eliminate this week?
Write it here:

....

Which new activity from page 125 are you going to include each
day? List them here:

Day 1: ....

Day 2: ....

Day 3: ....

Day 4: ....

Day 5: ....

Day 6: ....

Day 7: ....

Daily checklist	Day 1	Day 2	Day 3	Day 4	Day 5	Day 6	Day 7
Fat-Burning Pill	☐	☐	☐	☐	☐	☐	☐
First Affirmation session	☐	☐	☐	☐	☐	☐	☐
Second Affirmation session	☐	☐	☐	☐	☐	☐	☐
Visualising the future you	☐	☐	☐	☐	☐	☐	☐
Exercise Wheel	☐	☐	☐	☐	☐	☐	☐
The Lighten Up Diary	☐	☐	☐	☐	☐	☐	☐

My goal for the rest of the programme is:

....

....

CHAPTER ELEVEN

WEEK THREE
OF THE
EIGHT-WEEK
COURSE

HOW ARE YOU DOING?

You may have already noticed that reviewing your Diary and Challenges at the beginning of each week isn't a checklist exercise. You have your Weekly Checklist to remind you about the stuff that you want to do on a daily basis but the Diary and Challenges are different. You don't have to make sure you've checked off every single suggestion every week. Just go through them all and take a little time to think about them.

LAST WEEK'S LIGHTEN UP DIARY
AND CHALLENGES

Set aside some time to review your Diary and Challenges for the past week. The Lighten Up programme is all about getting to know yourself better and realising you can trust yourself to know how you feel and what you want. Noting the behaviour patterns and feelings revealed in your diary is a crucial part of this process.

★ What did the Exercise Wheel tell you about your exercise levels this week? Do you think there's room for more activity in your working day and your leisure time? You don't have to continue filling in the Exercise Wheel (unless you think it might be useful) but we hope it will have given you a good idea of where you are starting from.

★ What activities do you associate with eating:
   Working?
   Driving?
   Watching television?
   Reading?
   On the go?

★ How often were you able to eat without doing anything else at the same time?

★ How often did you eat for reasons other than hunger? And what were those other reasons that triggered you to eat?

★ How many times did you use the Hunger Scale?

★ How varied is your diet? Could you eat a wider variety of foods?

★ How was your food prepared? Are you eating most things fried? Or raw? Pre-cooked?

★ Do you think you are eating as much as you did last week?

★ Do you believe your Affirmation yet?

★ Is your visualisation becoming easier and more natural now? How strong is your image of the future you?

★ Are you noticing any patterns in your eating or snacking habits? Did you manage to change any of them?

★ How easy did you find it to use the Fat Jar? Did you manage it once a day?

Are You Ready?

★ Don't feel as though you should memorise everything we've worked on so far. Simply try out all the new techniques and ideas for the week as they are introduced and the Lighten Up Diary and Challenges at the end of each chapter will summarise what you should be focusing on this week. If you just stick with the programme, week by week, you will stay on track without even having to think about it.

★ However, if in the past two weeks you've discovered something you particularly like and which works well for you, by all means keep on doing it. This isn't a programme where you do something just once or twice and move on to something new. Similar techniques and ideas will be cropping up over and over again in different disguises, until you become totally familiar and comfortable with this toolbox for change.

WEEK THREE

In Week Three, as well as encouraging you to continue increasing your daily activity levels, we also want you to think about introducing some gentle exercise (Feel-good Fitness) for its own sake.

★ Calorie-saving Devices: why you need to increase your levels of everyday activity.
★ Fat Jar Fitness and Feel-good Fitness.
★ Back to Basics: guidelines for successful exercising.
★ The Whole Truth About the Whole-food Diet.
★ Eating Triggers: why you eat even though you're not hungry.
★ Your Relationship with Food.
★ Think Before You Eat: knowing what your body needs.
★ Eat for the Sake of Eating: getting maximum pleasure from your food and knowing when you're full.
★ Change: managing the changes that will help you slim.
★ Believe It and You're Ready to Achieve It: you *can* be slimmer.
★ Give Yourself Some Credit: tracking your triumphs.
★ Patterns: being aware of your own eating patterns.

CALORIE-SAVING DEVICES

Although we eat less than we did fifty years ago, we're also a lot less active so we tend to consume more calories than we burn. A Health Education Authority study showed that two-thirds of women aren't even active enough to be healthy. And it's not just hearts and lungs that are being neglected, it's bones as well. Our grandparents might not have gone to the gym three times a week, but they probably laboured for a living. Washing, cooking and cleaning were done the hard way and even social lives required effort in the days before cars, off-licences and videos.

Most people, when they look at their Exercise Wheel, are surprised by how much time they spend doing not very much. We drive to work, sit in front of the VDU all day, put the clothes in the washing machine, the dirty dishes in the dishwasher, buy ready meals and sit in front of the TV (for twice as long as we did in 1960), using the remote control. You may be *mentally* exhausted, but your body is bored.

Increase your daily activity levels

Some sad person calculated that you can burn an extra 132.3 calories a week by walking over to the TV five times a day instead of using your remote control. An even sadder person then objected that this was only true for people whose TVs were ten feet from their sofas. As you know, at Lighten Up we believe that calorie counting in general, whether it's calories in or calories out, is pretty futile. But these figures do make an important point.

We are encouraged to buy more equipment to save our energy. We are programmed to think it's a good idea to have lots of labour- and time-saving devices, which is fine if we're then going to do something exciting with all the time we've saved. It is, however, absolutely *not* fine if we end up spending even more of every day sitting down as a result. That's just bad for our bodies and, if our bodies aren't happy, our minds won't be either.

But it's easy to restore the balance – you simply need to increase your level of activity. One area where you could consider abandoning convenience in the interests of exercise is travelling. We often use cars and buses when we could walk or ride a bike and it sometimes doesn't make much difference time-wise. However, it will lose you pounds (and might save you pounds as well). Do what you've got to do, including washing up and scrubbing floors, with vim and vigour but bear in mind that there are far more interesting ways than this of being active. Once you've finished your chores, go out and do something just for fun like playing golf, cycling by the river, or taking your children for a swim at the local pool.

You wouldn't buy a dog and not bother to walk it, would you? So why treat your own body with less consideration than the dog? And if you haven't got a dog, that's no excuse – just buy yourself a pair of trainers and get moving.

FAT JAR FITNESS AND FEEL GOOD FITNESS

FAT JAR FITNESS

So far we've been talking about increasing your activity levels in everyday life – putting the coins in the Fat Jar every time you walk or cycle or vacuum the stairs. And this kind of exercise is vitally important because it's steady and continuous but comfortable. You're less likely to injure yourself – and you get some of the jobs done at the same time.

FEEL GOOD FITNESS[1]

But there's no harm in exercising for the sake of it as well – people have been fun-running since the first Olympic Games nearly three thousand years ago, and probably long before that. Grown-ups, sadly, lose their playfulness. I always feel sad when I'm in a health club and I see rows of people on exercise bikes, faces set in grim determination, working up a sweat just for the sake of it. Believe me, it doesn't have to be like that and it *shouldn't* be like that.

WHAT'S THE DIFFERENCE?

★ *Fat Jar Fitness* is just 15 minutes of continuous brisk activity. It's something you can do any time, anywhere and you

1 If you have been inactive for a while or you are trying something new, check with your doctor and then take professional advice on your chosen activity.

won't need to take a shower or put on special clothes to do it. And you can combine it with other activities. For example, a 15-minute walk might get you part of the way to work and 15 minutes flat-out housework could be very much like a fast walk with a bit of gentle weight lifting.

★ *Feel Good Fitness* is exercise that's worth doing for its own sake. It's something you do just for the fun of it like playing football or taking salsa lessons, but which keeps you fit and healthy as well. It's a bit more strenuous than Fat Jar Fitness, so you need to wear comfortable clothes to do it and take a shower afterwards.

DO YOU NEED TO DO BOTH?

If your job involves hard physical work, then you're getting the workouts at work and you're entitled to a sit-down in the evenings.

But if, like most people, your daily routine involves a lot of sitting down, or walking around quite slowly, you are going to feel much better if you combine your daily Fat Jar Fitness with some more strenuous weekly Feel Good Fitness sessions as well. Feel Good Fitness is an extra, a bonus, a gift you give yourself. See it as a bit of personal space in your life, time out to lavish attention on your body, your muscles, your health and your well-being.

So, now you're into your third week of the Lighten Up programme, it's time to consider introducing some regular Feel Good Fitness exercise into your life *as well as*, *not instead of*, the increased daily activity you are doing now.

MOVE IT AND LOSE IT

Make a note in your regular work diary or calendar to put in at least two Feel Good Fitness sessions this week. When you've done it, give yourself a gold star in your Lighten Up Diary.

Ideally, Feel Good Fitness should involve comfortable but vigorous exercise three or more times a week (though we're starting with just two sessions this week). Here are some ideas to make it easy.

Choose something you might enjoy and decide whether you want to be sociable or go it alone. It doesn't have to be circuit training or a workout at the gym. There are lots of alternatives so take into account your level of fitness, personal preferences and convenience, too. You're more likely to do something regularly if it's near at hand and easy to get started. It doesn't have to be expensive either – your Local Authority probably runs all sorts of evening classes in just about everything from t'ai chi to fencing.

Of course, you could buy a video or an exercise bike and work up a bit of a sweat in the privacy of your own home, using baked-bean cans for weights. However, we really don't advise you to start off that way. Why not? Because if you've been inactive for a while or you've never done much in the way of exercise before, you need to take some advice about the level at which you should be exercising and the kind of movements you should be doing. Everybody is different and you need to take into account your age, state of health and any injuries you might have sustained in the past. Joining a class or a group with a trained leader or instructor is always the best way to start.

Get a comprehensive list of what's available and get going. If you don't really enjoy your first choice activity, try something else until you find something that really suits you. Here are some ideas:

Aerobics	Martial arts
Athletics	Netball
Ballroom dancing	Pilates
Basketball	Power walking
Climbing	Rowing
Cricket	Salsa
Cycling	Squash
Fencing	Step classes
Football	Swimming
Golf (only if you walk	T'ai chi
briskly round the course	Tennis
and caddy for yourself)	Trampolining
Jogging	Weight training
Line dancing	Yoga

That's not a comprehensive list by any means. Just a few ideas to get you started, because getting started is the most important thing. Chapter Eighteen will give you a lot more detailed information about Feel-good Fitness.

The golden rule

Always stay within your comfort zone. If something doesn't feel right, don't do it. And don't set out to exhaust yourself and make yourself miserable. Remember the pleasure principle – make it work for you by finding ways to get pleasure out of everything you do.

Motivation

Here are a few motivational suggestions:

★ Set yourself a goal for every exercise session (e.g. *I'm going to feel refreshed and full of energy*).
★ Concentrate on what you're doing. Feel your body working. Watching television while you're on a treadmill may mean you're not maximising your training.
★ Think of yourself as sculpture – you are working on a fantastic piece of art (you!).
★ Listen to your body and work with it, not against it. If it hurts *don't do it.* Forget about going for the burn.
★ Incorporate some deep breathing into your routine. This alone will make you feel great. Breathe through your nose as much as possible.
★ If you watch someone take that first sip from a glass of wine, or the first nibble from a bar of chocolate, they often close their eyes and concentrate on the pleasure of the moment. Your brain is releasing similar chemicals when you exercise – so why aren't you taking notice?
★ Exercising with your mind on your body is a physical form of meditation. You will get so much more benefit from your workout if you focus your mind on what your body is doing.
★ If you want a better body, give the one you've got some consideration. When you're doing resistance training (working with weights), for example, be aware of the muscles you are working. Imagine the energy you're generating, imagine the

strength you're building, imagine those muscles the way you want them to be.

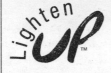 You get what you focus on while you're exercising too. So focus on what you want.

GETTING IT TOGETHER

Exercise, like eating, should be given the attention it deserves. Exercise is what your body was designed to do, and if you do it thoughtfully it will make you feel better. A lot of people behave as though using their mind and body together will somehow overload their circuits. They exercise because they think that working out to the point of exhaustion is the only way to lose weight. And when they've finished exercising and they switch their brains back on again, they notice that something hurts.

So they stop exercising for a while and get depressed and turn to food, or alcohol or artificial chemicals to cheer them up again.

I'm speaking from experience here. Working as a personal trainer, I've met a lot of these desperate slimmers and the fallout rate is high. But suppose they had been exercising *thoughtfully* in the first place? When you're aware of your body, you're more likely to spot the warning signs that tell you when to stop, when to ease up and when to keep going. You'll feel the injury before it happens – or at least before the damage is irreversible. And then you can take action to fix the problem and, meanwhile, vary your workout routine and give your knee (or your elbow, or your back or wherever the strain has appeared) time to recover.

STOP THE CLOCK

Exercising by the clock, without listening to your body, can lead to:

- ★ Boredom – you'll never do your best if you're bored. Reading a novel or listening to music while you exercise stops you focusing on the exercise itself, and you may even find yourself thinking 'I'd be enjoying this book a lot more if I were sitting in an armchair with a drink in my other hand . . .'
- ★ Under-exercising – you won't get the benefits if you exercise half-heartedly and you'll be far more likely to quit too soon or, worse still, quit altogether and drift straight back into that beer and pizza lifestyle.
- ★ Injury – you may miss the warning signs.
- ★ Burnout – if you aren't focused, you may exercise when your body's telling you not to. Maybe you've got a cold or you've been overdoing it lately – you could end up with long-term problems if you don't take the hint and rest.

MAKE TIME

There's a great deal of evidence that exercise does a lot more for your health than simply keeping you slim. Regular, steady exercise makes you less susceptible to all kinds of diseases, from colds to cancer. Saying that you can't find time to exercise is like saying you haven't got time to be healthy. Make yourself a priority. Make time for some regular Feel Good Fitness in your life – even if this means getting out of bed an hour earlier than usual.

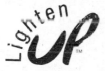 *These guidelines apply to Feel Good Fitness, the concentrated, intensive (but still comfortable) exercise sessions. They don't apply to whatever you're doing to fill up the Fat Jar. If you're doing a brisk Fat Jar walk (as long as you've got enough cushioning under the soles of your feet), you can let your body get on with it. That gives you time to look around you, think, plan, sing, talk to someone or listen to tapes on your Walkman. Or you could even be saying your Affirmations or practising some visualisations. It's only when you are exercising at the more intensive feel-good level that you need to be really concentrating on yourself and what you're doing.*

BACK TO BASICS

It all comes back to basics – the pleasure and pain principle.

We protect ourselves physically without even thinking about it. We flinch from a flying object, or jump back from something hot. It's a pity our psychological protection systems aren't as efficient. In fact, they can be downright dysfunctional. When we feel unhappy, do we react immediately and move away from the source of the pain? No. We're much more likely to intensify the problem by adding another piece of negative behaviour. Like getting drunk when we feel lonely or overworking because we feel insecure. It doesn't resolve the issue, it just distracts us temporarily and leaves us with more problems to deal with in the long run. It's like leaving your hand on the stove and taking morphine to kill the pain.

THE BIG BONUS

If you exercise regularly according to your body's capacity, you're going to enjoy it. Not only are you going to enjoy it, but you're going to *see* results – and that's a great reinforcer and source of pleasure. When you can see the change and improvement in your muscle tone or your stamina and strength, it's the greatest incentive in the world to keep up the good work.

I'm not saying that regular, thoughtful, concentrated exercise is the only way to be happy. But it's a great foundation – and the only side-effects seem to be good health and improved performance. Open your mind to the possibility of exercise for its own sake rather than doing it because you think you must.

Do yourself a favour: get up, get out, get moving and start feeling great!

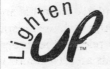

Lighten Up works because it covers what you do, what you eat and what you think. If you take away any one of these components, the scales won't balance.

So let's move on to our eating information for this week.

THE WHOLE TRUTH
ABOUT THE WHOLE-FOOD DIET

One of the best ways to stay slim and healthy is to eat food that doesn't have a label on it listing loads of ingredients. The best food for you is *unrefined*. It's been grown and sent to the shop without going via the factory. Be curious about what you're putting into your body. If you don't know what it is, the chances are it's not good for you.

YOU ARE WHAT YOU EAT

We are organic living creatures and we need food that is as fresh as possible. Although our bodies can use processed or refined food, we won't get the best nutritional value from it. A study by the National Heart Forum in 1997 estimated that more than 30,000 lives could be saved in Britain each year if everybody ate at least five daily portions of fruit and vegetables.

A lot of the food we buy is refined to give it a longer shelf life without losing its taste. This sounds sensible enough in theory, but in practice there are some downsides to eating it.

★ The refining process can break down the food into simpler forms so that it's digested very fast, sending a lot of glucose very quickly into the bloodstream, which can cause problems for some people. There's more detail about this in Chapter Seventeen.

★ Some of the nutritional value is lost during the refining process, which means that eating a lot of these foods can cause vitamin and mineral deficiencies.

★ Refined foods, like cake, chocolate, biscuits and soft drinks, provide energy but lack nutrients, particularly vitamins and minerals. This creates a problem because the body needs specific vitamins and minerals in order to release the energy from food. If those vitamins and minerals aren't present in the food itself the body has to raid its existing stores of them.

It's hardly surprising that these refined foods are called 'anti-nutrients' – they are robbing us of some of the essentials of life.

★ As if that weren't enough, refined foods tend to contain a lot of artificial additives and many of these substances just haven't been around long enough for us to be certain they're harmless.

 Just take a look at the ingredient lists from three very commonplace foods you'll find on any supermarket shelves. Can you guess what these products might be?

1 Maltodextrin, food starch, vegetable fat, flavourings, hydrolysed protein, tomato powder, salt, sugar, colours (E150, E1240), dried oxtail, dried beef, beef fat, flavour enhancer (monosodium glutamate), citric acid E330, antioxidant (E320, E321).

2 Pork, chicken, water, beef, vegetable protein, dried skimmed milk, salt, spices, sodium tripolyphosphate (E450C), antioxidant: ascorbic acid, preservative, sodium nitrate.

3 Sugar, wheat flour, water, cherries, vegetable fat (with antioxidant E231), dried glucose, syrup, modified starch, skimmed milk powder, cheese powder, gelling agents (E327, E339, E450), sodium caseinate, emulsifier (E472B), stabiliser (E401), salt, fumaric acid, citric acid (E330), flavourings, preservative (E211), colours (E102, E122, E124, E142, E151).

(1. Packet soup; 2. Sausages; 3. Shop-bought cherry cake)

We are omnivores, which means that, like pigs, we'll eat any old rubbish and generally survive on it. In fact, it's probably the key to our survival as a species. If our diet were as limited as the giant panda's or even the koala's, it's unlikely that we'd have populated as much of the planet and multiplied at the rate we did. Humans can eat anything from whale blubber to bugs and get by. But however tolerant our bodies are, there's overwhelming evidence that we do better on fresh, natural foods.

Unfortunately, because we've learned to eat for reasons other than hunger, we've formed strong associations with sugary, salty foods that are easy to eat when we aren't hungry. A lot of these snacks are full of chemicals (which our bodies have had only a few years of learning to tolerate) as well as sugar, fat and salt. Perhaps the genetically modified human beings of the future will do very well on the food that is toxic to us right now. But for the moment we are still fairly primitive organisms as far as food is concerned and we flourish on a fairly primitive diet.

MINOR CHANGES IN YOUR EATING HABITS CAN LEAD TO MAJOR CHANGES IN YOUR SIZE, SHAPE AND STATE OF HEALTH

You are the most sophisticated piece of equipment with the most powerful and intelligent software that you'll ever own. Once you learn to acknowledge your body and give it what it needs, it will work much better for you.

 Nutrition is a serious subject, but food is still fun. Take a look at the recipes in the back of the book and try out something new today. Make it something you wouldn't normally cook. Be adventurous!

EATING TRIGGERS

Knowing what you need to eat to keep you healthy is all very well, but actually doing it is a different thing altogether. In theory, realising you are hungry and that what you need is a banana is pretty straightforward. In reality, popping out of the office for a minute because the pressure is getting to you and walking past the bakery just as they're putting the doughnuts in the window is probably a more likely scenario.

 So, what are your triggers for overeating? Tick any of the following that looks familiar:

Parties   Boredom
Restaurants   Frustration

Eating alone	Fear
Eating with friends	Tiredness
Buffets	Mornings
Weddings	Afternoons
Diets	Being at work
Christmas	Holidays
Your Birthday	Summer
Congratulating yourself	Winter
Comforting yourself	Insomnia
Loneliness	Feeling fat
Stress	Depression
Cooking	Anger

FEELING FED UP

Lots of things trigger us to eat and the list above contains just a few examples.

The more eating triggers you have, the fatter you probably are. The key is to learn to eat only when you are hungry and to do something different when you're not. We'll be talking about alternatives to eating when you aren't hungry in Week Five, but the key is to find something that meets the same need. For example, if you eat because you're bored, the obvious alternative is to do something interesting like reading a good book or going shopping. Or if you eat because you're lonely then you could think about joining in with more social activities.

Maybe you're triggered to eat by the desire for pleasure because so many people associate pleasure with food. Or perhaps it's comfort, or reassurance, or support . . . When you're upset, the first, most familiar suggestion your helpful subconscious mind might come up with is 'how about something salty, sugary or just plain fattening to cheer you up?' But you don't *have* to say yes to everything your subconscious suggests. You can politely ask it to come up with another alternative. And if that doesn't work, say something a little stronger, like 'shut up!'

Whatever it is that makes you turn to food when you aren't hungry, it's just a habit you've learned, practised and mastered. Congratulations. The question is, are you ready to change it?

DO THIS NOW Name and shame, right now, an eating habit you want to get rid of. Give yourself permission to live without it – permanently.

YOUR RELATIONSHIP WITH FOOD

Relationships with food can be complex. That's why it helps to keep the Diary – it's the story of a relationship that's making you unhappy. But like most difficult relationships, you need to understand it before you can do anything about it.

We use food for comfort, food to celebrate and food to console. Different events, feelings, times and trigger situations can make us feel like eating, regardless of whether or not we're hungry. Seeing food, or even pictures of food (which are everywhere), smelling food, seeing somebody walk past with a hamburger. Even looking at the clock. There's no escape from the suggestion that it might be time for something to eat.

Many of the foods we eat in these situations are fattening ones that leave us feeling tired, bloated and guilty. When we ask ourselves afterwards 'why did I eat that?' it's too late.

But help is at hand: at Lighten Up we've talked to lots of slim people and discovered that almost all of them have one thing hard-wired into their brains that overweight people don't. It's a mental technique called Think Before You Eat and it's one of the most important tools for becoming slim and staying slim.

It's very simple: you just get into the habit, before you eat, of stopping to think what food options you have and imagining how they would taste and smell and how you would feel after you'd eaten them. Most naturally slim people have their own version of it. It's something I've always done myself and Connirae Andreas describes a similar process in her book *Heart of the Mind*.

Although naturally slim people usually stop and run through a range of possibilities before they make a choice, people with weight problems often have a much less selective eating strategy. They can be triggered to eat by a time of day, an activity, a feeling, an event, a person, a place – anything, in fact, other than hunger.

Thinking Before You Eat doesn't always work immediately. Like the other techniques in this book, you can do it alone or with a friend. Whichever suits you. It takes a few minutes to get to grips with at first but with a bit of practice you'll be able to zoom through it in seconds. Take it seriously, though, it's a powerful piece of software for reprogramming your mind and body.

THINK BEFORE YOU EAT

Something makes you think of food. You might look at your watch and notice that it's lunchtime, you might hear the word 'chocolate', or see someone eating a bag of chips. Or you might even feel hungry. So:

 Find a quiet place where you can relax. Ask someone to read this exercise out to you (or record it yourself on to a tape). Close your eyes.

★ Now that the idea of eating has come into your mind, check whether you're getting any physical sensations or perhaps you could just be lonely or bored.

★ If you've got some feelings that make you think you are over 5 on the Hunger Scale, ask yourself what your body actually needs.

★ What comes to mind? A double hamburger with melted cheese? A banana? A slice of chocolate cake? Some foods are easy to imagine (think of biting into a lemon) but anything that doesn't give your tastebuds a tingle is probably not something you really want at all.

★ Now run through the process of eating it in your mind. Taste it, smell it, feel it in your mouth and swallow it. Imagine how you'll be feeling half an hour and then an hour afterwards. What do you imagine this food looks like inside your body? What colour is it? Does it give you energy or make you feel tired?

★ If you think you'll feel better once you've eaten whatever it is than you do now, put the item on to a mental list. However, if you don't think whatever it is will see you happily through the afternoon don't bother to make a note of it.

★ Keep doing this until you've got a few choices in mind.

★ Check out your choices, one at a time, for their long-term effect on your happiness and well-being.

★ If you find it difficult to distinguish between 'good and satis-fying' and 'naughty but nice', try a few deliberately wacky opposites. Like toffee crunch ice-cream with treacle tart com-pared with a tuna salad sandwich on granary bread.

When you get fed up with doing this (or your lunch break is run-ning out), make a decision. Most people find, over time, that this process leads them away from the obvious choices of highly refined and heavily overpackaged foods towards more natural, healthy options.

The aim of this exercise is to put you back in touch with what your body truly needs. If you actually give it a chance it will guide you towards the foods that are good for you rather than the foods you're used to, or those that are just easy to get hold of and eat.

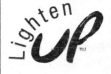 *Stop fighting with yourself and start listening. You'll free up a lot of energy, which can be directed into things that make you feel happy and in control instead of miserable and out of control.*

EAT FOR THE SAKE OF EATING

Eat for the sake of eating? Can we be serious? Yes, we are – all too often we eat while we're concentrating on something else. Use food like a drug to ease your pain and it becomes a bad habit – a quick fix, rather than a lingering sensual pleasure.

Since I've been working with Lighten Up, I've spent a lot of time watching other people eating. Family, friends, clients, strangers in restaurants. In fact, there was a time when I was probably North London's least popular dinner companion.

What did I notice – apart from the fact that nobody likes to be watched while they're eating? I noticed that the people who ate the most enjoyed it the least.

Big eaters are often fast eaters. Dieters typically spend a great deal of time between meals thinking about what they are allowed (or not allowed) to eat next. But then they swallow the food they allow themselves in a few minutes, almost without noticing it. It's often not what they really wanted to eat, or when they wanted to eat it anyway.

We're asking you to be aware of every mouthful you take. Enjoy every single one, instead of trying to get through it as fast as possible and then suffering a lot of guilt afterwards – over something you never even tasted.

Eating can be an automatic process, often done without much appreciation. If you think you sometimes (or often) eat without thinking about it, you may be missing out on:

★ signals that tell you you're full
★ the kind of foods your body really needs
★ the pleasure of eating.

KNOWING WHEN YOU'VE HAD ENOUGH

Take time over your meals. Even something as simple as chewing your food more slowly will slow down your mealtimes and give your stomach more time to register when it's full.

Our stomachs contain sensory nerves that tell us when to eat and when to stop. It takes a while for the brain to get the 'I'm full' message from the stomach, so give it time and listen.

WHAT YOUR BODY NEEDS

Concentrate on the taste and texture of what you're eating. Smell it first and see how appetising it is before you even put it in your mouth. If you're at a buffet or in a canteen, take time to separate out the smells before you make your choice.

Don't ever decide what to eat by appearance alone. Always (discreetly) sniff the food first. And if all you've got is a menu, close your eyes and use your imagination. You'll be surprised by how often your first automatic choice is contradicted by your nose.

Smell is the sense that links most directly to the brain and it's your sense of smell that will help you to get back in touch with what your body really needs. This approach is likely to lead you, over time, to make some surprising choices and it will guide you back to a varied and well-balanced diet.

ORGASMIC EXPERIENCES

Eating's important enough for you to give it your full attention. It's one of the greatest sensual pleasures of life, so why rush it?

See just how much pleasure you can get from your food. Set aside time to eat when your mind isn't somewhere else. And enjoy.

Once you make your eating a focused, orgasmic experience, you'll get much more pleasure from it, as you resensitise yourself to the signals your body naturally gives out – signals that you might have been ignoring for some time.

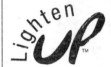 *You'll find that eating this way will also give you a much better understanding of how food makes you feel.*

Pick one of the following and do it at least twice a day for the next week:

★ See just how much pleasure you can get from your food. Set aside time to eat when your mind isn't somewhere else and your body isn't doing something else – and enjoy.

★ Share a meal with someone else, provided you agree to focus on the sensual pleasure of eating. Remember the meal in *Tom Jones*? If not, get it out on video and you'll see what we mean.

★ Put your knife and fork down between mouthfuls and leave them on the plate for at least 30 seconds.

★ Take the serving dishes away from the table so you won't be tempted to eat more simply because it's there.

The concept of eating for its own sake can sometimes stop a meal before it even starts! Often, if you eliminate the activity you associate with eating and just sit down to eat, you'll find you aren't even hungry – it was simply the association with that other activity that made you think you were.

If the idea of eating slowly bothers you, it's probably a sign that you are hooked on the association of eating with other activities. It's a cliché, but the harder it is to do, the more you need to learn to do it.

POINTLESS EXERCISE

Eating when you aren't hungry is a pointless exercise: your body won't use the food to produce extra energy and make you feel good, it will just store it as fat. Have you ever said 'I feel fat' when you've overeaten? That's because you're absolutely right.

CHANGE

You can do almost anything you put your mind to, but first you need a strong, positive, long-term goal. Your brain will work towards whatever it is you're focusing on. And since most people focus on what they want to avoid, it's not surprising that that's exactly what they get.

Take weight, for example. People tend to spend more time thinking about the weight they want to lose than about how good they'll look when they've lost it. We spend more time worrying about things that could go wrong than anticipating good times ahead. *Looking forward* is something children do before Christmas and birthdays. *Worrying about what might happen* is something adults do all the time.

My friend Lisa once said, 'There's no point in looking forward to something nice – you don't need to practise having fun, do you? It's the horrible things you keep going over in your mind because you hope by doing that you'll be able to cope when the worst happens.'

I remember getting really cross with her. 'Honestly, Lisa, have you ever wondered why you don't enjoy parties and holidays as much as you used to? You're the world's expert at expecting the worst, so it's hardly surprising that it's what you usually get. You wouldn't want to waste all that preparation, would you?'

Surprisingly, she's still talking to me.

The most popular TV programmes are the soaps – the more catastrophes per hour, it seems, the higher the ratings. We are all fascinated by misfortune – but then we wonder why we're feeling so anxious and pessimistic.

It's the same with weight. Many overweight people tend to think about their extra pounds all the time and the body generally follows what's in the mind. If you are starving or over-exercising your body while your brain is still playing the 'fat person' video, of course you're going to fail.

Why not start planning for success? If disasters happen, you'll cope anyway. It's success you need to plan for. Once you've practised some positive anticipation a few times, your brain will have a much clearer idea of where you want to go.

 All the greatest achievers of the twentieth century, from Edison to Branson, started by being successful in their minds. Remember when you used yourself as a role model in Week One? Take a moment now to think about some other things you did in your life that involved positive changes, large or small, and start a list in your Diary.

MAKING A HABIT OF CHANGE

Change isn't always easy, but it's definitely *possible* with determination and the right help; which is what this book is for, of course!

Attempts to change usually meet the strongest resistance at the beginning. Your body protests when you first drink tea without sugar. Then, after a while, the tea doesn't taste right with sugar in it. Sometimes other people don't like you changing either. If you say no to a HobNob, they might feel guilty about eating one themselves. But once you get over the first hurdle, you're likely to succeed.

Many of our eating patterns have been with us for years. We've been comforted, placated and rewarded with food since we were too small to argue. We're taught to associate food with emotions from our earliest days. But no matter how long we've been doing this, it's not something we were born with, and the good news is that we can change. We don't have to be stuck with any of those learned behaviours. With strength and determination we can unlearn them and install some new and more empowering patterns.

Most of us prefer an easy, predictable life. If change seems hard, it's not so much because of fear of the unknown as our desire to stay inside our comfort zones. Lighten Up encourages you to break out of your comfort zone and take action to change your habits. It's worth remembering that, as we mentioned in Chapter Nine, people who've succeeded in becoming slimmer usually associate pain with inactivity and overeating, but considerable pleasure with being active, fit and slender.

Can you control your perception of what is pain and what is pleasure? Of course you can. But you can only start the process by taking decisive action and it may be a bit uncomfortable to begin with. The challenge is for you to *use* pain and pleasure instead of pain and pleasure using you. That's the secret of success. If you do this you will be in control of your life. If you don't, then life controls you.

MORE STRENGTH TO YOUR ELBOW, AND KNEES AND ANKLES AND SHOULDERS . . .

Practise becoming stronger and more flexible. Every time you make the decision to do something positive like walking to the shops, trying a new form of exercise or cycling when you'd normally take the car, you are becoming stronger and more able to cope with change.

Change is happening in and around us all the time. We grow new cells, we learn new ideas, the seasons turn and the weather is never what you expect. So open up to change and changes will happen.

 Clasp your hands so that you have one thumb on top of the other. Don't think about it, just do it. Now look at which thumb is on top. Unclasp your hands and clasp them again, but this time put the other thumb on top. How does that feel? Most people find it strange. Well, that's change for you: it feels a bit uncomfortable – but you can do it. Do this 20 or 30 times, each time with a different thumb on top and you'll eventually find it's becoming quite comfortable either way.

A CHANGE PROCESS

The techniques and ideas in this book aim to teach you how to use your mind and body to get what you want. If you have the desire then you also have the ability to take action. If you use the exercises that are right for you, you can be slimmer for ever.

Some people are born with advantages: a powerful, healthy physique, money, a supportive family and great educational opportunities. Maybe, you might say, some people are born thin. But there are plenty of people who didn't start out with any of those advantages and they still ended up looking good, feeling great and attracting as much love and money as they wanted.

How did they do that? They did it by making committed decisions about what they wanted and following those decisions with action for change.

 Answer these questions, either in your head or in your Lighten Up Diary.

Questions:

Do I expect to achieve my goals?

Can I see myself looking like and feeling like the person I want to be?

Can I turn that image of myself looking and feeling good into a movie with me as the star?

If the answer to these is 'yes', go on to make the Affirmation.

If the answer is 'no', you have two choices:
1 Keep working on your beliefs until you get a clear strong 'yes', or,
2 Stay as you are and like yourself that way.

Affirmation: *I am getting slimmer.*

Decision: *I know that staying slim means leading an active life and eating a healthy, varied diet. I know what it takes and I'm already doing it.*

BELIEVE IT AND YOU'RE READY TO ACHIEVE IT

Once you've put some effort into *believing* what you want, the effort you need to *achieve* it will seem relatively straightforward.

Do you believe you can be slimmer?

Whether you believe you can or believe you can't, you're right. It's up to you to pull your own strings. All the effort and energy you put into being slimmer won't necessarily get you there unless you really believe it's possible. The function of your brain is to confirm what you believe. So if you believe you're fat, stupid, or you can't do something, you're right.

It's worth considering what other strong beliefs you have.

War is a bad thing
The sun rises every morning
Exhaust fumes are damaging our environment
Being slimmer will make you feel better
Life's a beach and then you fry
Love is wonderful

You weren't born believing any of those things, you simply picked them up as you went along. That's how beliefs are formed. You will have plenty of references as to why you believe in something; maybe it was something your parents told you, you read about it, you discussed it and now you believe it. Sometimes we hold on to beliefs built on references that are obsolete, outdated or outgrown.

Perfectly intelligent people have been known to live their lives thinking they were completely stupid, solely on the basis of random remarks their teachers made. Yet beliefs which are strong enough to limit our lives and make us unhappy often have the flimsiest of foundations.

Beliefs are just rules and generalisations we've made for ourselves. How can we ever know which are valid and which aren't? How do we know which to live by and which to abandon?

 Think of a negative belief you have about yourself and ask yourself how you know it's true. Could you let that belief go? Right now?

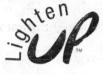 *If your beliefs serve you well, if they help you to become slimmer, fitter, healthier, happier and more confident, then they are good ones to have. But if your beliefs are making you unhappy, dysfunctional and fat, bin them.*

GIVE YOURSELF SOME CREDIT

A great way to reinforce your belief in your ability to be slim, and stay slim, is to give yourself credit whenever you deserve it. The Great British Upbringing teaches us to focus on our faults and failures, while modestly ignoring our triumphs. We learn this from a very early age and it's a sure recipe for low self-confidence and poor self-image.

So, it's time to redress the balance.

Remember the exercise in Week One, when we suggested you could be your own role model and learn from your past achievements? Well, now it's time to go a step further and recognise your own day-by-day and minute-by-minute achievements instead of letting them slip by unnoticed while you worry about the failures.

 for the rest of your life:

★ Whenever you score a hit in the Diary, for enjoying a meal, knowing when you're hungry or going for a walk instead of downing the seventh pint, congratulate yourself.

- ★ Give yourself a big smile whenever you put a coin in the Fat Jar.
- ★ Do your daydreaming practice at regular intervals. See yourself doing good things and accepting recognition for them gracefully.
- ★ Give yourself a pat on the back whenever you catch yourself doing something right and the Diary isn't at hand.
- ★ Give yourself positive messages regularly during the day. Encourage yourself as you go along. Now that you're in the habit of repeating Affirmations to yourself regularly, this kind of self-reinforcement will come a lot more naturally.
- ★ Be kinder to yourself and give yourself permission to make mistakes.

If you recognise the good things that happen and constantly look out for them, you'll find more and more of them tend to come your way.

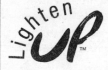 *Take responsibility for tracking your own triumphs. And remember, size really doesn't matter. Acknowledge the small triumphs as well as the earth-shattering ones.*

PATTERNS

Remember Mo? The girl who reformed her Kettle Chip habit so successfully? Well, I saw her at a wedding the other day and when the cake came round she simply waved the plate away. I took a piece myself and, when I turned back, I saw she was grinning like a Cheshire cat.

'What? What's funny? And why didn't you have any cake?' I asked her. 'Is it because you didn't make it and you don't think it's up to standard?'

'No, it's not that at all. I didn't want any – and now, when I say "no" to something I don't want, I feel so pleased with myself, I'm kind of cheering in my head at my own achievement. And that makes me feel even better.'

It didn't even occur to me to laugh at her for congratulating herself over a piece of cake. How could I – after the time we'd been through a few years ago when her weight seemed to be the only thing in her life she couldn't control and the one thing she cared about more than anything. I wish more people would give themselves this kind of credit. Congratulating yourself is the best way I know of making good behaviour stick, yet most people rely on others to tell them when they're doing well.

Successful people are different: they are much better at recognising their own achievements.

We live in a society focused on problems and the possibility of things going wrong. We're programmed to expect failure and often don't notice when we do get something right.

But from now on, instead of reliving every defeat and disaster, you're going to make a mental note of every time you do something right, or even write it in your Diary. Keep the memory handy for an action replay when you need a boost.

After all, we all like to be told when we do something well. The trouble is, we can become completely dependent on other people to give us that feedback – and feel let down when we don't get it. If you congratulate *yourself* whenever you deserve it, you need never miss out again. And it might take the pressure off your nearest and dearest because you won't be depending on them for support and encouragement all the time.

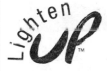 *Recognising your own behaviour patterns is a really easy behaviour pattern to acquire. And it's self-reinforcing – once you start, it's hard to stop.*

THE LIGHTEN UP DIARY

New Notes
★ Make a note of every meal you eat without doing anything else at the same time, and whether you eat as much or less than you normally would.

★ Make a note of every time you run the Think Before You Eat exercise before a meal and how helpful it is.

Carry On writing down
★ what you eat and drink and when;
★ what triggers you to eat;
★ where you are on the Hunger Scale;
★ how eating makes you feel and what feelings make you eat;
★ what food tastes like;
★ how much of your food is refined or processed and how much is fresh food. Look at Chapter Seventeen if you want to know more.

As you write, keep looking for patterns and make a note of one you get rid of.

CHALLENGES

★ Add in at least two Feel-good Fitness sessions this week.
★ Eliminate another unwanted eating pattern.
★ Slow down your eating.
★ Use the knife and fork rule (you don't have to time the 30 seconds exactly!) and taste every mouthful.
★ Take the serving dishes off the table so you aren't tempted to keep picking just because the food's there.
★ Spend time every day visualising yourself looking and feeling the way you would ideally like to be. The way you would look on Oscar night if you'd been nominated for best actor. Assume that you have a limitless budget and a couple of months to prepare. Remember – you get what you focus on.
★ Tell yourself a hundred times a day that you expect to be slimmer.
★ Take at least one more Fat-burning Pill so that you are getting two fifteen-minute sessions of Fat Jar Fitness every day.
★ Cook something new from the recipes in Chapter Nineteen.

CHECKLIST FOR WEEK THREE

Weekly checklist

Which eating pattern are you going to eliminate this week?
Write it here:

....

On which two days are you going to do your Feel Good Fitness
sessions? Write them here:

Feel Good Fitness session 1: ....

Feel Good Fitness session 2: ....

Daily checklist	Day 1	Day 2	Day 3	Day 4	Day 5	Day 6	Day 7
First Fat Burning Pill (Fat Jar Exercise)	☐	☐	☐	☐	☐	☐	☐
Second Fat Burning Pill (Fat Jar Exercise)	☐	☐	☐	☐	☐	☐	☐
First Affirmation session	☐	☐	☐	☐	☐	☐	☐
Second Affirmation session	☐	☐	☐	☐	☐	☐	☐
Open Door exercise	☐	☐	☐	☐	☐	☐	☐
Congratulating yourself on an achievement	☐	☐	☐	☐	☐	☐	☐
Thinking Before You Eat (Morning)	☐	☐	☐	☐	☐	☐	☐
Thinking Before You Eat (Noon)	☐	☐	☐	☐	☐	☐	☐

continued

Daily checklist (continued)	Day 1	Day 2	Day 3	Day 4	Day 5	Day 6	Day 7
Thinking Before You Eat (Evening)	☐	☐	☐	☐	☐	☐	☐
The Lighten Up Diary	☐	☐	☐	☐	☐	☐	☐

My goal for the rest of the programme is:

....

....

CHAPTER TWELVE

WEEK FOUR
OF THE
EIGHT-WEEK
COURSE

HOW ARE YOU DOING?

The Diary isn't about what you eat or what you're supposed to eat. I'm not asking you to write it all down so you can criticise yourself. The reaction to what you write should be: *'Hm, that's interesting, there's a pattern there . . . I wonder why I do that? Would I like to change that? What else could I do?'* Don't start weeping over the page or calling yourself names because you ate too many Jaffa Cakes. It doesn't matter. They're eaten. List them and let them go, and next time you eat a Jaffa Cake, *enjoy* it.

However, if you notice that you seem to be putting rather a lot of ice-cream into your Diary, the question you need to ask yourself is: 'What would be the most enjoyable way of turning this fat into fuel?' Then go and do it. ASAP!

The Lighten Up Diary is about being aware of what you do. There's a saying in management training: 'If you can't measure it, you can't manage it.' It applies to eating just as much as it does to building multi-billion-pound corporations.

LAST WEEK'S LIGHTEN UP DIARY
AND CHALLENGES

So, having said all that, how *did* you get on with writing every-thing down last week? Was it easy to make a regular note of what you ate? If not, what stopped you? Embarrassment often tops the list here and, if your eating embarrasses you, isn't it time to start being a bit more honest? The other reason people give for not keeping their Diary is that they couldn't be bothered.

My answer to that is: 'How much does being overweight bother you? – What's it worth to make a change?'

When you look through your entries for the week, are your eating patterns predictable, or surprising? Usually you'll find some of both. I've asked a lot of questions below, but it's worth taking the time to go through them slowly and think about the answers. They are important to you. (Writing down the times you eat is easier if you keep your Diary as you go along.)

★ Does your eating cluster during certain parts of the day?
★ Does it vary according to the day of the week?
★ Do you eat more at weekends?
★ Did you succeed in changing one dysfunctional eating pat-tern last week?
★ Have you noticed some changes happening already? Can you make a list of them in the Diary?
★ What do you notice about the taste of your food?
★ Are you enjoying your food more or less than you did before you started on the programme? Are you noticing anything about the way certain food tastes to you now?
★ How many meals did you manage to eat without doing any-thing else at the same time? And how did that feel? Did it affect the amount you ate?
★ What level are you at, typically, on the Hunger Scale before you eat?
★ What about the feelings that might have been making you eat when you weren't really hungry? Have you discovered whether you eat when you're depressed, happy, anxious, angry, lonely? If you find yourself eating at less than 5 on the

Hunger Scale, run a quick check for the presence of one of these emotions – or whatever the feelings are that make *you* fall into the comfort-eating trap.

★ Were you aware that sometimes you might be eating when you weren't really hungry?
★ How was Think Before You Eat? Are you starting to do it automatically yet?
★ Is food making you feel good? Or is there still a bit of residual guilt around?
★ Did you manage to slow down your eating? Did putting down your knife and fork and moving the serving dishes make any difference?
★ How much processed and pre-prepared food are you eating and how much fresh food?
★ How easy did you find it to encourage and congratulate yourself every time you did something really well?
★ Are your Affirmations convincing you yet?
★ Are you still focusing on what you want to achieve, what you'll look like and what you'll hear and feel? Did you do the Open Door exercise from Week One every day last week?
★ How clear is your picture of yourself – the way you would *like* to be?
★ How confident are you of your success?
★ What are you getting out of being more active?
★ How full is the Fat Jar?
★ Did you manage to add in those two Feel Good Fitness sessions last week? How did they make you feel?
★ Did you try a new recipe?

Are You Ready?

This week marks the halfway point in the Lighten Up programme and you may notice that some changes are starting to happen. They may be dramatic or they may be subtle but it's often around this time that people begin to feel that their patterns of eating and exercise are more controllable than ever before.

If you were taking part in a Lighten Up workshop I'd be telling you to make yourself and your well-being a priority for the next few weeks. So go ahead and do just that. Put yourself first, give yourself the time and space you need to think through these ideas and test out the suggestions. Then use your Lighten Up Diary to give yourself the feedback you need.

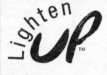

WEEK FOUR

This week we'll be talking about the two main anxiety generators in the world of slimming: how much to eat and how much to exercise.

★ On a Scale of 1 to 10: The Borg Scale[1] will show you how to exercise at the right rate for you.

★ Fat Jar Fitness and Feel-good Fitness: getting more of both into your life.

★ The Lighten Up Food Profile: this is a very important part of the Lighten Up programme. It's important because it helps you to get a better idea of whether you are eating well and what you might be missing. But it still isn't rules and it isn't a diet.

★ Sugar: the secret saboteur.

★ Outcomes: the stepping stones towards your goal.

★ Lapsing, Relapsing and Collapsing: knowing the difference.

★ There's No Such Thing as Failure: the Success Formula.

ON A SCALE OF 1 TO 10

How much more active have you been over the past few weeks? Do you realise that you're getting fitter, slowly but surely? Every minute you exercise and every step you take is turning you into a more efficient fat-burning machine.

The secret of staying slim is to eat sensibly and take plenty of exercise – hardly a revelation, you might think. But people always look very disappointed when we tell them that. Surely it

1 Named after the man who invented it.

can't be that simple? If it's so easy, why do 95 per cent of people who diet (instead of Lightening Up) still fail?

We'll start this week, as usual, with the exercise side of the equation because it's exercise not dieting that changes your body chemistry so that you can burn more fat than ever before. The more active you are, the more fuel you'll burn, even when you're resting. The main criterion for weight loss is that the exercise you take should be comfortable; continuous and steady – but comfortable.

There are as many mixed messages about exercise as there are about diet. It's a bit like the veggie versus carnivore battle. It's hard to convince a dedicated couch potato that his neighbour is really cycling to work by choice. And the jogger, dependent on his daily endorphin high, pities the flabby commuter gasping for breath as he heaves himself on to the train at the last minute.

So who's right?

There are undoubtedly some troubled souls who exercise beyond all need or capacity. Either they don't have much of a home life or they really enjoy being taped up to that ultrasound machine when they've injured their leg for the fourth time that year. But there are also people who love to move and exercise, but who know that, if it hurts, it's not doing them any good.

How do you change the minds of the thousands of people who are convinced that exercise is going to hurt? Who believe that the only reason for doing it is to burn as many calories as possible and get it over with. The idea of enjoying it for its own sake is incomprehensible to them.

Take another step closer to your ideal future self by making these your exercise goals:

★ Staying healthy
★ Teaching your body to burn fat
★ Feeling good for no good reason
★ Having fun

Now, doesn't that sound good?

Fat is the energy source we use while we're sleeping, sitting, working and even eating. Fit people are efficient at using it and fat people are efficient at storing it. Exercise is the key to turning a fat-storing body into a fat-burning one but the important thing is to enjoy the process itself. Expect to feel those endolphins[2] swimming around your body and making you feel fantastic.

The Borg Scale

More scales (in case you were getting withdrawal symptoms)! This is a very simple scale to help you judge for yourself whether you're exercising at the right level.

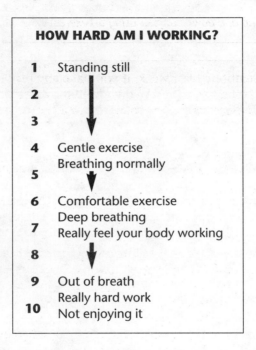

The Borg Scale works on the same principle as the Hunger Scale and, like the Hunger Scale, most people react to it the first time by saying, 'Yes, but how do I know whether I'm at 6 or 7?' We tell them, 'Just behave as if you know.' And they go away and do it. Like a lot of the techniques we use, the Borg Scale involves

2 I may be dyslexic, but I do know how to spell endorphins. I just think endolphins sound more fun.

asking yourself questions. While you're exercising, ask yourself what level you're working at and grade it 1–10. Ideally you should aim for 6–7–8 for a period of 15 minutes to one hour. Make sure it's comfortable and continuous.

Experiment to find out how hard you have to work to reach the various levels; get familiar with your own heart and breathing rates and how they vary. You can do this simply by walking up and down stairs or using an exercise bike.

As we mentioned last week, if you have any medical problems or if you haven't exerted yourself for a while take your doctor's advice before you change your activity pattern.

Aerobic exercise should always be comfortable, regardless of your level of fitness. If you can't talk or whistle at the same time, you're overdoing it. If you're hating every second and feeling totally out of breath, it's because your body is failing to get oxygen to your muscles. When that happens you're working without oxygen, that is, anaerobically.

Muscles need oxygen to function and the harder they're worked the more oxygen they need. But hard doesn't mean painful. Aerobic exercise simply means exercise that uses oxygen. Feel Good Fitness is definitely aerobic exercise and if your Fat Jar Fitness involves quite vigorous activity like really brisk walking then that is aerobic too. The difference is just a matter of degree. We've differentiated between the two because we are trying to get across the message that it's not just the intensive kind of exercise (Feel Good Fitness), which needs a change of clothes and a shower afterwards, that is good for you. Lower intensity, everyday activity (Fat Jar Fitness) will also build muscle and improve your cardiovascular fitness, but you need both.

Why? Because for most of us in sedentary jobs the acceptable level of everyday activity is unlikely to involve us using our bodies as much as we were designed to do. It's a lifestyle thing that comes with plumbing and deodorant sales – it's just not acceptable for a human being who's been sweating hard to spend a day at a desk next to another human being.

So we suggest that you maintain a steady base level of fat-burning activity with your Fat Jar Fitness, while boosting your muscular and aerobic fitness with regular sessions of Feel Good Fitness.

In order for the body to burn fat, it needs a large amount of oxygen. However, if you exercise so hard you get out of breath you won't be getting enough oxygen and your body will be working too hard. Remember, the body needs oxygen to burn fat. If you're seriously out of breath you're burning sugar, not fat.

 Give yourself five minutes and find a quiet place. Work through the following sections on Fat Jar Fitness and Feel Good Fitness. Write your responses in your Diary.

FAT JAR FITNESS

We'll start with your everyday activity levels – because, as you know by now, Fat Jar Fitness, or making exercise part of your daily routine, is a basic requirement if you want to stay slim. Any Feel Good Fitness exercise you do is a bonus.

The secret is to sneak activity into everyday situations whenever you see the slightest opportunity: run up the stairs, walk up the escalator, walk to work, get a basket on your bike and cycle to the shops, throw away the remote control and walk over to the TV, walk to a local that's not quite so local and, if you're thinking of buying a pet, make it a greyhound, not a goldfish.

How can you include even more activity in your daily life?

★ Walk to work.
★ Cycle to work.
★ Walk at lunchtime.
★ Get into the habit of starting or ending the day with a 15-minute walk. If you like *A Book at Bedtime*, or music in the morning, take it with you on a Walkman.

I commit to being more active by including the following activity in my daily life:

....

....

Signed ....

FEEL-GOOD FITNESS

'I'm too busy' is the most common reason people give for not exercising. But they're not too busy to watch TV or go to the pub. The only way you'll ever make exercise part of your life is if you learn to enjoy it. Keep your bigger, long-term picture in front of you, so you're constantly aware of the benefits of your exercise routine. If your goal is to become fitter, slimmer and healthier, and to have loads of energy and vitality, what sort of role will exercise have in your vision of the future? Focus on how your Feel Good Fitness routines will give you energy, keep you healthy and release any tension or stress.

★ What do you want to achieve?

....

★ What part does exercise play in achieving it?

....

★ What do you want exercise to do for you?

....

★ What are the benefits you get from exercising? How does it make you feel?

....

★ What would it cost you if you didn't exercise at all?

....

★ How can you make your exercise even more enjoyable? Below are some suggestions but you may have a completely different solution:
- Partnering with a friend to maintain your interest and motivation.
- Joining a gym.
- Working with a personal trainer to personalise your routines – this works well if you're an impatient personality and you want instant results.
- Finding new ways of exercising.
- Buying a piece of exercise equipment for your home.
- Taking up a sport.
- Using an exercise video.
- ....

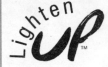

Movement, activity – exercise, call it what you want – is the only way to become successfully slimmer forever. Exercise educates your body to burn fat.

THE LIGHTEN UP FOOD PROFILE

On page 191 is the Food Profile. For the next five weeks – and longer if you want to – you'll be marking everything you eat on a copy of these two circles. The Food Profile is going to help you see how healthy and balanced your diet is now and how much more healthy and balanced it's going to become.

The Foods to Focus On in the top circle are the ones you want to make sure you get plenty of, and the Foods to Limit in the bottom circle are the less healthy foods that you might want to eat less of.

But it's all food and it will all keep you alive. The difference is that the Food to Focus On will not only keep you alive, it will also keep you slim and healthy. The important thing is to be *aware* of what you're eating and make sure that you're getting *enough* of the really good stuff.

The Food Profile is not an eating bible, it's a way of tracking

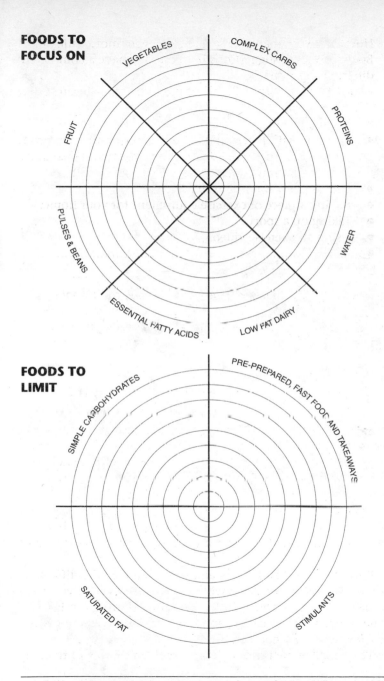

FOODS TO FOCUS ON

VEGETABLES
COMPLEX CARBS
FRUIT
PROTEINS
PULSES & BEANS
WATER
ESSENTIAL FATTY ACIDS
LOW FAT DAIRY

FOODS TO LIMIT

SIMPLE CARBOHYDRATES
PRE-PREPARED, FAST FOOD AND TAKEAWAYS
SATURATED FAT
STIMULANTS

your progress. It's not meant to be totally comprehensive or perfectly consistent because we don't want you to start using it like a set of rules. In fact, having paid quite close attention to what you eat over the past few weeks, we now want you to move away from focusing on your food in such minute detail. The Food Profile is a rough guide to show you that you're moving in the right direction with your eating patterns. If you try to be detailed and precise with it you'll come unstuck.

Nutrition is a highly complex science and that's not what Lighten Up is about. We want you to eat when you're hungry, take more exercise and choose the kind of food that will do you good. The Food Profile is designed to help you do that, it won't be accurate to the letter *but it will give you a very good idea of how you're doing*.

Chapter Seventeen gives you much more detail about the Food Profile, together with lists of foods which will help you know which categories to use. And if you want to know a little more about the nutrition behind it, Chapter Seventeen also has more information on this. But, just to get you started, here's the basic information you need.

DO THIS **from now on:**
Make a copy of the Food Profile for every day, stick it into your Diary and put the date at the top. Every time you eat or drink something, put a cross in the appropriate section of one of the circles. You probably have a pretty good idea of which circle your food fits into, but if you're not sure, simply check the more detailed lists of foods in Chapter Seventeen.

Each morning, start in the middle of the circle and work outwards with each serving. Some segments will fill up faster than others. If you reach your outer circle, just draw some more circles round the outside.

WHAT WILL THE FOOD PROFILE DO FOR YOU?

The Food Profile is specially designed to help you make sure you're getting a varied diet. It's not a formula, it's a guide to a slimmer, fitter you.

DO THIS NOW

At first glance, have you noticed anything in Foods to Focus On that you might be short of? Make a mental note, or a note in your Lighten Up Diary to include whatever this is on your next shopping list. In fact, this would be a good time to *start* your next shopping list and your Diary might be as good a place as anywhere.

This isn't about denial or deprivation, it's about meeting your body's needs for health, strength and fitness. If there are some healthy foods you simply can't bear, find substitutes that fall into the same category. Perhaps some new recipes would help – take a look at the recipes in Chapter Nineteen if you feel in need of inspiration.

A lifetime of food denial punctuated by occasional bingeing is a miserable way to live – but it does serve the need for self-punishment that a lot of us seem to have. Most people on diets are aiming to cut out the binges – eventually. But of course they can't, because their bodies can only take so much of the pain and denial and, sooner or later, the yearning for pleasure (albeit the guilty pleasure of a binge) becomes unbearable.

Some diets actually use this principle to their advantage by offering you a system which lets you binge on certain food groups while cutting others out altogether. This provides pleasure and pain at the same time. However much cabbage soup or red wine or grapefruit you're allowed, you're bound to yearn for the sausages and overripe bananas you're not supposed to eat. Diets like this are unbalanced and can cause deficiencies in vital nutrients.

A happy balance is the key to healthy eating, but you're going to have to start being nice to yourself if you're going to achieve it.

FOOD IS YOUR FRIEND

Food isn't the enemy. Unless we eat the right amount of the right food our bodies can't function properly. Food is energy, it's fuel, it's essential. Not eating is always fatal, and starvation and malnutrition kill at least as many people as overeating and unbalanced eating.

THE FOOD PROFILE WILL KEEP YOU ON TRACK

The Food Profile is your eating reference for the next five weeks. And that is all it is – a reference, *not* a set of rules. There are plenty of limitations to it if you want to look for them – just fill it out as best you can and see how your eating patterns change. The bottom line is that the more of your eating there is on the top circle and the less on the bottom circle, the slimmer and healthier you are going to be.

This is not a strict regime or a complicated formula, it's just a simple, visual way of seeing whether you are eating a healthy, balanced selection of food every day. By using the Food Profile you can steadily lose weight, while at the same time ensuring you're eating a good balance of foods from different food groups. The Food Profile works on the principle that you need a little of everything and that too much of anything will turn to fat – even if it starts out as skinned chicken breasts and steamed spinach.

HOW DO YOU KNOW WHAT YOU'RE EATING?

Some foods are straightforward. If you have a banana, or a glass of water – or even a cup of tea with two teaspoons of sugar – you know exactly where to put your crosses. But it's more difficult to keep track of exactly how many servings of what to fill in when you're living on pre-prepared and fast food. Which is why we've made it easy for you by giving you a Pre-prepared, Fast Food and Takeaways section. Just put the whole meal in this section each time you have one of them (I'm afraid you have to disregard any healthy bits of tomato that might be balanced on top of your kebab) and keep an eye on how many processed meals you're eating over the week.

We haven't included restaurant meals in the Pre-prepared, Fast Food and Takeaways section because in many restaurants there are healthy options and you have more choice about the way your meal is put together. But make your own decision on this – if you're eating in at your local hamburger chain, then the cross had better go in Foods to Limit.

BEWARE . . .

★ Those processed, ready-made meals and takeaways we just talked about can be full of saturated fat, sugar and additives, and low in nutrients.

★ Beware of low-fat 'diet' products. They are often higher in sugar than their 'normal' alternatives and they're usually full of chemicals.

★ If you eat anything containing fat *and* sugar together, such as chocolate, cakes and biscuits, it's highly likely you'll blow your fat and sugar servings in one go. If you assume that four small biscuits contain all your saturated fat and sugar for the day, you'll start to get a clearer picture.

★ Did you know that one Mars bar contains eight teaspoons of sugar? So be smart with cakes, biscuits and confectionery. If you fancy a little, have a little, but make sure the rest of your food that day contains no added fat or sugar.

THE DEVIL'S IN THE DETAIL

Don't try to be precise. Just as we don't want you weighing and measuring everything, you don't have to fret about whether you've filled in your daily Food Profile down to the last gram. If you've eaten a meal that doesn't seem to break down into anything that fits the categories, just mark up what you think the closest category is.

HOW MUCH IS ENOUGH?

How much you need to eat depends on your body's individual needs. The only way to gauge this is to get to know yourself and that's what the Hunger Scale, Think Before You Eat and the Lighten Up Diary are all about. Get used to the idea of observing yourself without being critical. And while you're getting properly reacquainted with yourself (yes, you did know all this once, you've just forgotten) you can use the Food Profile.

Don't try to get it exactly right. It can be very difficult to work out precisely how much of everything you should eat, so don't bother – it's not necessary to be that accurate. Of course, most diets do tell you exactly what to eat and how much because its easier than learning to work it out for yourself. But unfortunately learning to trust your own judgement is the only way to stay slim in the long run. The Food Profile is a guide to what types of food you should be eating for life – but only *you* will know how much. And you will know by listening to your body and learning to eat when you're hungry and stop when you're full.

You can waste a lot of time weighing out rolled oats and counting beans. If you really must have a ritual, make it Think Before You Eat, not weights and measures. And if you've still got time on your hands and food on your mind, try the What Do You Want? exercises in Chapter Seven, either alone or with a friend. Start getting to know the slimmer, happier you. Practise your Open Door exercise until you have a bright, clear, compelling image of how you could look and be. You'll soon find it's difficult to eat the kind of food your body doesn't need at times when it's not really hungry.

Look for balance. As you start to respect your body more, give it more of the foods it really wants and listen to the response. Let your body tell you when it's hungry and when it's full.

Make gradual changes and enjoy what you eat.

SUGAR – THE SECRET SABOTEUR

There's a lot of information about different food groups in Chapter Seventeen. But during the Lighten Up course we will spotlight a few of the issues we think are particularly important.

We start with sugar. Fat is usually the biggest, baddest bogey in the slimming world but, in fact, sugar is just as much of a problem. It's part of the carbohydrate group, but because it's the simplest form of carbohydrate it's lacking in a lot of the good things other carbohydrates have – like fibre and vitamins and minerals. And because it's so quickly absorbed and you get such a fast hit from eating it, it's also addictive. Anything that's addictive is potentially a problem for a lot of people.

What foods are you most likely to crave? What food do you instinctively reach for when you're lacking energy? We're all sugarholics sometimes and you might be interested to know that there are now a number of studies highlighting the dangers of eating too much sugar.[3] The powerful sugar industry is widely blamed for the fact that, until recently, many of these studies haven't been given much publicity.

There's an alarming amount of 'hidden' sugar in prepared and processed foods. Even so-called healthy foods, particularly the ones with low-fat labels, contain lots of sugar. A well-known breakfast bran cereal, for example, is 22 per cent sugar and a famous slimming meal-substitute drink is 61.9 per cent sugar – higher than many brands of sweet biscuits and cakes. In fact, slimming foods, as we've mentioned before, often contain a great deal of extra sugar to compensate for the fat which has been taken out.

SWEET AND HIGH

It's not just drugs that give you the feel-good-feeling rush we all crave. Sugar does it too. Answer these questions to see if you might have a problem with sugar:

	Yes	No
I can live without cakes, chocolates, sweets, soft drinks or biscuits.	☐	☐
I can go for a day or so without eating any of those things.	☐	☐
I can always stop after eating one sweet or biscuit or a single piece of chocolate	☐	☐
I can have a cupboard full of sweet snacks and not eat them.	☐	☐
I rarely drink soft drinks.	☐	☐
Coffee, cereal, strawberries and raspberries taste better without sugar.	☐	☐
I'm usually too full to want anything sweet at the end of a meal.	☐	☐
There are times when I don't have any sweet treats in the house.	☐	☐

If you answer 'no' to three or more of these questions, you may well be sugar sensitive.

3 Dr William Grant, NASA, 1999, Jack Winkler, Cyndi Thomson, Mary Whiting, Linda Lazarides, Michael Lean.

No one claims sugar is the sole cause of being overweight, but sugar and salt are the two tastes everybody reacts to instantly – you can always eat something sweet or salty, even after a big meal. Which is why most snacks are high in one or the other (and some have both!). Of course, too much salt also causes health problems, so the simple answer is to eat as many natural foods without added salt or sugar as possible.

SWEET COMFORT

Have you ever come home after a long, hard day, feeling tired and a little hungry. Maybe not very hungry, you're not sure, but you want something. There's nobody around to talk to. What do you do? An awful lot of people in that situation will reach for the chocolate, the biscuit or the piece of cake. It's easy, it's comforting and it's quick.

YOU ARE PROBABLY SWEET ENOUGH

Has anybody ever said 'I'm sweet enough' when you asked them if they wanted sugar in their tea? Maybe they really meant, 'I'm happy enough – I don't need sugar to cheer me up.'

GUIDELINES FOR CUTTING OUT SUGAR

★ Gradually cut down on the amount of sugar you add to food and drinks.

★ Buy reduced or sugar-free versions of food and drinks, like sugar-free baked beans, but check that they don't contain any artificial sweeteners as there is some evidence they may not be good for you.

★ When you're baking you can often use a lot less sugar than the recipe suggests. Sometimes you can even halve the amount – or substitute fruit or fruit juice. Fruit contains sugar but at least it's not empty calories.

★ Beware of anything ending in 'ose' on food labels. Some foods may have up to four or five different types of sugar in them. But they are all sugar.

★ Check your food labels. You'll be surprised at how much and how often sugar sneaks into food.

- ★ White grapes and dried fruits are excellent for staving off sugar cravings. They're high in sugar, but also in nutritional value.
- ★ Choose foods which are sweetened with juices or fruit, so that at least you get the vitamins as well as the sugar.
- ★ Visit your local health shop. They have loads of healthy sweet treats. But be cautious, as they also have loads of unhealthy sweet treats. Always check the labels, even in health stores.
- ★ When you have the urge for something sweet, ask yourself, 'Is this hunger or a craving?' If it's a craving, do something else. Cravings come in waves, they build up and die down. Ride the wave.

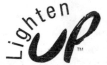 *The first few weeks of this course have focused more on your goals than on the details of food and nutrition. Which is why we've only just introduced the Food Profile and started talking about sugar. We want you to get the message about sugar and be cautious about it. But at the end of the day it's a detail. And getting bogged down in the detail of dieting is exactly the reason why so many people fail to lose weight.*

So, let's get back to the big picture of a smaller you in the not too distant future.

OUTCOMES

You're probably wondering why we're talking about outcomes now when we were talking about goals in the last few chapters. Yes, there is a difference. Of course, outcomes and goals are just words. They can mean the same thing if you want them to, or they can mean nothing at all if you don't bother to set them, review them and follow them up.

You started the Lighten Up programme with a specific goal, the one you wrote down in Week One. Since then we've been encouraging you to work on that goal to make sure it takes account of the changes in your life, and still inspires and motivates you. If you think about your goal and visualise it every day it will become clearer and more real and compelling to you; it will feel like part of a plan that's already under way rather than just a dream for the future.

That goal is your destination and if you want to reach your destination you have to plan your route. Outcomes are the mini-goals, the short-term daily objectives that provide you with the stepping stones on the way to your final objective.

For example:

★ Today I am going to get most of my crosses in the Foods to Focus On circle.
★ Today I am only going to eat when I'm more than 6 on the Hunger Scale.
★ Today I am going to cycle to work and walk up the escalators.
★ Today I am going to workout for 20 minutes and put five pence in the Fat Jar as well.
★ Today I am going to give myself credit every time I do something positive.
★ Today I am going to spend five minutes visualising myself being even slimmer, fitter and healthier.
★ Today I am going to feel good and release any stress.

DO THIS NOW Set yourself a couple of outcomes for the rest of today. They don't have to be slimming ones – it's up to you. Just make them positive.

....

....

If you want to enter them in your Diary, go ahead.

Once you've got into the habit of setting and achieving your outcomes, you're quite likely to turn into a success junkie. You'll want to keep achieving and succeeding. The buzz you'll get from taking one successful step after another towards your ultimate goal will create its own momentum.

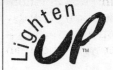 *If you don't manage to achieve today's outcome, find out why, learn from it and do something different next time.*

SCORING GOALS

The goal you set yourself may change as you work your way through the Lighten Up programme. But that's fine, it's like sailing a boat: as the tide and wind conditions change, you adjust to keep yourself on track. Adjusting and resetting your outcomes on a daily basis makes the process seem very much more manageable. If you like you can make this very easy for yourself by making the weekly Challenges your outcomes and simply following them on a daily basis.

By setting and achieving outcomes, you'll also get into the habit of experiencing success. If you want to get more out of your daily life, start setting yourself outcomes for everything you do.

For example, if you are going out with some friends, ask yourself, 'What do I want from this evening?' If you were to set yourself an outcome like 'I'm going to have a good time and enjoy myself', then that's what you are going to get. You get what you focus on. On the other hand if you said to yourself 'I hope I don't get drunk and eat too much . . .' that's what might happen.

Suppose you were to ask yourself 'What do I want to get out of today?' You might set yourself an outcome like: 'eating when I'm hungry, taking my Fat-burning Pills and having some fun'. If you commit to doing this, then that's what you are going to get.

 Pause for a moment and set some outcomes – some steps towards your ultimate goal – right now:

What do you want to have achieved by this time tomorrow?

....

What do you want to have achieved by this time next week?

....

Write them down in the Diary.

Think of the feelings you get when you accomplish some-thing. Even the feeling you get when you tick an item off your 'to do' list. It doesn't matter whether it's cleaning out the fridge or completing your first novel. You'll get the same good feeling whenever you achieve an outcome, and feel the satisfaction of taking positive action that is making you slimmer, fitter and healthier.

LAPSING, RELAPSING AND COLLAPSING

Setting daily outcomes, or stepping stones towards your goal, will not only make sure you arrive at your destination in good condition; they'll give you something to hang on to when you have a lapse. And even if you relapse or collapse.

What's the difference? Lapses and relapses are nothing to worry about. They're just behaviour patterns.

Collapses are more serious because they are based on beliefs, not behaviour.

A *lapse* is a slight error or slip, a little backslide. It's a one-off event, like eating crisps and peanuts all night at a party, or a whole tub of ice-cream one lonely evening at home, or getting up too late to walk to work for a few days. It doesn't matter. Once it's done (or not done) it's over with. *This is when you have the unique opportunity to learn. You don't need to make the same mistake again.*

A *relapse* is when you manage to string together a whole series of lapses so that it starts to look like the state you were in before you started changing. *Even in this situation you have the capacity to change things. Remember, it's up to you, no one else is involved. It only takes a second to change. Be willing to do whatever it takes to get your outcome.*

A *Collapse* happens when you start believing your old nega-tive beliefs about yourself again. It happens when you feel it's not worth bothering to change any more. Or when you find you get just as much satisfaction from whining about your weight as you would from being slim. *If you think you're having a collapse, then this is the time to reflect on what happened and how or why it happened. But don't pause for too long. Instead turn things around and start again with the benefit of hindsight. You can use the success formula on the next page to turn any perceived failures into successes.*

THERE'S NO SUCH THING AS FAILURE

Edison was given the finance to make an electric light bulb, an idea which had been the despair of inventors for 50 years. It took him 14 months of trial and error to find a suitable filament and he got it wrong hundreds of times before he finally got it right. But every time he tried an unsuitable material he merely took the view that he had eliminated yet another possibility and was therefore one step closer to finding a permanent solution to the challenge.

There is an old saying that 'a path with no obstacles goes nowhere'. There are always going to be times when you make a mistake or think you've failed. Most of us fear failure because we think it means that *we* are failures. But failing is just something you have to do occasionally – it's the other side of success. When we get things wrong, it's an ideal opportunity to learn.

What you've done is less important than your response to what you've done. So if, for example, you overate because you were stressed, or tired, or bored, just say, 'OK, that's what I did this time – what will I do differently next time?'

Think back to when you learned to drive or ride a bike. You almost certainly didn't get that right first time. But the mistakes you made were signposts that gave you the opportunity to learn.

Dieters are always one mouthful away from failure: one piece of chocolate or a late-night binge and they think, 'I've blown it.' What a great excuse to dive back into your old bad habits. But once it's eaten, it's finished, it's history. Stop beating yourself up and get on with your life. The successful slimmers I've worked with have used experiences like this as opportunities to learn. Keep learning.

THE SUCCESS FORMULA

Think of the last time you lapsed or failed in your efforts to be slimmer. Perhaps you snacked when you didn't need to, or even binged for a few days. Maybe you went away for a fortnight and neglected yourself for the whole time (by not exercising, not drinking enough water and not eating healthy food, perhaps). It could be a major blip, or just a tiny one.

 Go back to the last time it happened and talk yourself through it again.

Step One   Notice yourself

- making a mistake;
- talking to yourself in a self-defeating way;
- giving yourself a hard time.

Step Two   **Stop**. Pause and halt the process for a moment.

Step Three   Talk to yourself constructively, encouragingly.

Step Four   Become curious about what made you behave the way you did. Laugh at it. The behaviour isn't important. Your response to it is what matters.

Step Five   Ask yourself some useful questions: 'What, specifically, triggered me to behave this way? What started the overeating or the chocolate binge? What was I thinking about just before I did it?

Step Six   When you understand why you did what you did, ask yourself: 'What will I do differently next time it happens, so that I get a different outcome – one that doesn't involve eating?'

Step Seven   Consider the alternative courses of action:

- go for a walk;
- phone a friend;
- have a bath.

Step Eight   Come up with your own strategy: if you don't learn from your mistakes, you'll make them again.

Step Nine   Look, learn and move on.

Success is on the other side of failure.

THE LIGHTEN UP DIARY

You're probably learning some interesting things about how your feelings and state of mind affect your eating patterns. Seeing things written down in black and white often makes you notice things you missed before. And, as you become more and more aware, you will also start to feel much more in control of your eating.

New Notes

★ Now that you have the Food Profile, you can stop writing down everything you eat and drink and just put crosses in the circles instead. It should save you a lot of time and free you up to use your Diary more creatively instead of just making lists. Copy the Food Profile seven times, once for each day of the week, just as you did with the Exercise Wheels and fill it in every day. But remember, you can't carry foods forward to the next day, or spread one day's virtuous eating over a whole week. If you eat enough spinach for seven days on Monday, you'll just be wasting it. There won't be enough room to fill it in on Monday's chart and your body isn't going to get more than one day's benefit from it either.

★ Make a note of when you include some foods that you consider to be particularly healthy, especially if they are quite new to you. Do you enjoy them? How do they make you feel afterwards?

★ Every day write down the outcomes that will lead you to your ultimate goal.

★ Notice and write down when (or if) you have cravings for sugar. If you are deliberately eating less sugar at the moment, is that having a positive effect or a negative effect on how you feel?

★ Watch out for any lapses in the Lighten Up programme (or relapses, or collapses) and use the success formula to put them in perspective. Describe how it works.

Carry On

★ writing down what triggered you to eat – hunger, boredom, stress or any of the other usual suspects;
★ where you were on the Hunger Scale each time you ate;
★ feelings associated with food. How food makes you feel or, perhaps, what makes you feel like food.

CHALLENGES

★ Add an extra Feel Good Fitness session so that you are doing three sessions a week now. It doesn't have to be the same kind of exercise as the others and, if you didn't enjoy what you were doing last week, you could always try something completely new.
★ Use the Borg Scale to make sure you are doing your Feel Good Fitness exercises comfortably and effectively.
★ Eat at least two meals a day without doing anything else at the same time. Pause between mouthfuls and concentrate on enjoying every bite.
★ Change another negative eating pattern.

CHECKLIST FOR WEEK FOUR

Weekly checklist

Which eating pattern are you going to eliminate this week?
Write it here:

....

On which three days are you going to do your Feel Good Fitness
sessions? Write them here:

Feel Good Fitness session 1: ....

Feel Good Fitness session 2: ....

Feel Good Fitness session 3: ....

Daily checklist	Day 1	Day 2	Day 3	Day 4	Day 5	Day 6	Day 7
First Fat Burning Pill	☐	☐	☐	☐	☐	☐	☐
Second Fat Burning Pill	☐	☐	☐	☐	☐	☐	☐
First Affirmation session	☐	☐	☐	☐	☐	☐	☐
Second Affirmation session	☐	☐	☐	☐	☐	☐	☐
Open Door exercise	☐	☐	☐	☐	☐	☐	☐
Congratulating yourself on an achievement (however small) before you go to sleep at night	☐	☐	☐	☐	☐	☐	☐
The Lighten Up Diary – your first week with the Food Profile	☐	☐	☐	☐	☐	☐	☐

My goal for the rest of the programme is:

....

WEEK FIVE OF THE EIGHT-WEEK COURSE

HOW ARE YOU DOING?

You're Lightening Up for the fifth week, which means you're more than halfway through the course! You're probably noticing that you're taking more exercise than you've been used to. And you can imagine how it will feel to be even more active by next week.

Of the changes you made last week, which was the easiest? Was there something that fell into place so naturally you wondered why you'd never done it before? And were there any changes you really had to struggle with? What changes do you wish you'd made last week? Could you be able to make them this week?

What surprised you most about last week? It may not be directly to do with eating. Although we are beginning to talk more about food as the Lighten Up programme progresses, what still matters much more than what you eat is how you treat yourself. In a word: self-respect.

RESPECT

If you respect your body and your own good intentions, you're much more likely to succeed, whether it's in losing weight or winning a game of tennis. When you respect yourself, you're more likely to eat what your body needs and exercise regularly, and you're more likely to have a positive self-image to work towards.

So forget about calling yourself names and start giving yourself more credit. It's one secret ritual you can be proud of and you can substitute it for the nightly weigh-in, now you've got rid of your scales.

LAST WEEK'S LIGHTEN UP DIARY AND CHALLENGES

★ How did you get on with the Food Profile?

★ Where are you on the Hunger Scale when you eat?

★ Did you deliberately add any healthy foods this week?

★ Have you been setting yourself outcomes that will help take you closer to your ultimate slimming goal?

★ Are they working out? And are you setting up ones you really *want* to aim for – or ones you think you *ought* to aim for?

★ If you have any problems with sugar cravings, have you been keeping track of that this week?

★ How have you been dealing with any lapses you may have had over the week?

★ Are the same things still triggering you to eat? Did you manage to change another negative eating pattern this week? Are you getting clearer and more in control of the feelings that are associated with food for you? When you look back over your Diary, not just for this week, but for the past four weeks, how many changes have you made?

★ How was your extra Feel Good Fitness session? Have you decided what you want to do for the time being or are you still experimenting with different kinds of exercise? Is the Borg Scale helpful?

★ Is the Fat Jar filling up?

★ Are you using the Think Before You Eat strategy every time you eat?

- ★ How were your Affirmations? Have they changed at all?
- ★ Did you run the Open Door exercise every day? How do you find it now that you've been practising visualisation for the past few weeks?
- ★ Did you find something to congratulate yourself about every night before you went to sleep?

Are You Ready?

This is the stage when you Lighten Uppers sometimes get a bit too comfortable – you're starting to see changes by Week Five and it's easy to take it all for granted. So this is a good time to review where you are, look back over the Diary so far and do some intensive visualisation.

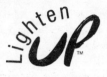

WEEK FIVE

This week we get down to some pretty basic stuff – eating and breathing! There isn't so much detail about exercise, but we hope you'll be popping a Fat Burning Pill at least a couple of times a day and doing three Feel Good Fitness sessions every week.

- ★ The Movie: polishing up your self-motivation.
- ★ Overfed and Undernourished: the importance of some of the key food groups.
- ★ How to Be a Breatharian: conscious breathing exercises to keep you calm and focused.
- ★ Good Times: finding some pleasure fixes.
- ★ Displacement Activities: distracting yourself from eating when you aren't hungry.

THE MOVIE

Do you remember the Open Door exercise? And the Affirmations you've been saying to yourself every day since Week Two?

We're hoping that both the Affirmations and the Open Door exercise will be feeling quite natural and easy to you now.

Visualisation is one of the most powerful ways of building yourself a compelling future that you can turn into reality. Sally Gunnell used this technique to help her win her Olympic gold medal. She practised seeing, hearing and feeling what it would be like to win until it became so real that she felt she had no choice but to succeed. You can do exactly the same with your slimming goal.

 Here's an opportunity to practise visualisation again and put your Affirmation to good use at the same time.

★ Imagine a picture of yourself in the future when you are as slim, fit and healthy as you want to be. You could be on a beach or at a party, or trying on some new jeans that fit you perfectly.

★ Imagine two more snapshots of yourself achieving a goal – they could be exercise goals, work goals or personal ones. It doesn't matter as long as they are clear and vivid.

★ Spread the images out in front of you.

★ Now sit in your imaginary director's chair and take the first image, the one of you looking so slim, and project it on to a huge screen right in front of you.

★ Look at that image for a moment, then pull up the second picture and project that on to the screen so that you can look at it properly. Finally, put the third picture up on the screen and give it your full attention. Take the time to notice what it is about these images that make them so compelling and attractive to you.

★ Now run those three experiences together as a film. They may be totally different, but it doesn't matter. Make a movie out of them, on that screen in front of you, and remember it's in technicolour with surround sound.

★ Now, step into the movie. And as you step into it, say your Affirmation to yourself.

★ Run the movie from start to finish with yourself as the star, trying on the jeans, lying on the beach or doing whatever it was you were doing in the original pictures you made.

★ See what you would have seen and hear what you would have heard – are people talking to you? What can you feel? Are there any sounds or feelings that make the experience more intense? And could you focus on those feelings even more than you are doing now?

★ When you've finished, run the film again, but this time, you are back in the Director's Chair, watching your performance.

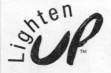 *Always run the film first with yourself on the inside, acting in it. Then sit back and watch it. If you do it that way round, your conscious mind is powerless to argue.*

OVERFED AND UNDERNOURISHED

This week we'll be focusing on the Food Profile and asking you to think about whether you're getting the foods you need now that you're more active. It may seem strange to be talking about whether you're eating enough on a slimming programme, but it is quite possible to be overfed and undernourished. Many children who live on chips and sweets are suffering from precisely this problem. So I'm going to be devoting a lot of page space to food groups and hints on eating a healthy diet.

You're going to be spending more time than usual this week thinking about what you eat as well as more time actually eating it. Thinking about what you eat is only a temporary stage in the Lighten Up process: we'll be focusing on it for the next couple of weeks, but as we said last week, after this we want you to spend the rest of your life enjoying food, not worrying about it.

OVERTIRED AND UNDERACTIVE

The right kind of carbohydrates won't change your life and neither will any particular combination of food groups. However wonderfully balanced your diet, if you want to stay slim your activity levels matter at least as much as your calorie levels.

One thing we notice about most new Lighten Uppers is that they often seem tired. At the beginning of a new eight-week course the energy levels in the room are usually pretty low. Sometimes it's because people are carrying a lot of weight – but not always. Some of the people who join the groups aren't extremely overweight – they're just exhausted by their lifelong battle with food.

One of the most common complaints you hear from people nowadays is that they're overtired. But we're physically doing less than we've ever done before and our grandparents didn't take as many holidays as we do. The problem, of course, is inactivity. Inactivity tends to make you lethargic. And the more lethargic you are, the less active you are, and the less active you are, the more fat you accumulate and the less you feel like exercising . . .

By this stage – Week Five – in a Lighten Up group, the energy levels are usually starting to rise. Everyone is feeling more optimistic; they are seeing clearer pictures of a brighter future and, of course, they are becoming a lot more active. The more active you are, the more energy you'll have to burn. And you know where energy comes from: **food**.

Raw energy

OLD WIVES' TALES?

The first thing most people notice when they fill in the Food Profile is that they aren't getting enough fruit and vegetables. We don't recommend fruit and vegetables because they're all low in calories – some are and some aren't. We recommend them because they're generally a much better source of vitamins and minerals than any amount of vitamin pills and supplements.

Carrots help you see in the dark[1] and broccoli makes your hair curl.[2] Maybe, maybe not. But the old saying that people who eat their greens will grow up to be big strong boys (and girls) is true. The propaganda machine for vegetables started

1 Yes.
2 No.

rolling during the Second World War when meat and sweets were rationed and expensive, and the government was trying to put a positive spin on cabbage and turnips. It wasn't until later that the health services looked at their statistics and realised the hype had proven spectacularly true. During the years of rationing there was a marked fall in heart disease, high blood pressure and diabetes.

Opticians didn't go out of business and neither did hairdressers, although the pressure on a lot of GPs' surgeries certainly eased. But right now, instead of a choice between a couple of apples or no pudding, we have 52 flavours of ice-cream to decide between.

Science is constantly researching the link between plenty of fresh, natural fruit and vegetables and good health. The American Institute for Cancer Research estimated in 2000 that as many as 40 per cent of all cancers in men and 60 per cent of those in women are linked to poor diet.

Humans are natural, organic creatures. We are not made of additives, chemicals or preservatives. Our bodies naturally want fresh, healthy fruit and vegetables to keep us full of health, energy and vitality.

Fruit and vegetables

HOW GREEN IS YOUR FOOD PROFILE?

If you are one of the majority of people whose Food Profile isn't yet registering enough of the green (or red, or blue, or yellow, or orange) stuff, don't despair.

A lot of people don't eat enough fruit and vegetables because they think they're boring and time-consuming to prepare. That's not true. And you will find, as you increase your daily intake, that the more and greater variety you eat of them the better they taste. Fruit and vegetables are also a great way of filling yourself up healthily – eat them whenever you're hungry. Vegetables and salads respond well to a little planning and creativity but you don't have to be vegetarian to make them a very enjoyable and major part of your diet. And remember – variety is the spice of life.

DO THIS NOW

So why *don't* you eat enough fruit and vegetables? (If your Food Profile is looking pretty well-balanced, skip this by all means.)

Did you have traumatic childhood experiences with dodgy fruit and soggy, over-cooked vegetables?

Try some completely different ones and cook them in more interesting ways.

Were you *forced* to eat fruit and vegetables as a child because they were good for you?

Experiment with fruit that's exotic so it seems more like a sinful luxury. Buy a juicer and make your own drinks. You can buy ready prepared fruit and vegetable juices, but beware of sugar and other additives.

Fruit and vegetables are too messy to eat while you're working or travelling?

If you want to be slimmer, it's not a good idea to eat on the go. It's easy to overeat when you're doing something else at the same time so it's better to make fruit and salad and vegetables a basic part of your main meals. But if you insist on snacking at your desk or in the car, there are lots of ways to do it:

★ Choose fruit with peel, like bananas and oranges, then you don't have to worry about washing or wrapping them up.

★ Prepare some fruit, raw veggies, salad or soup in the morning, put it in a plastic box or a flask and take it with you (plus a spoon).

Are fruit and vegetables too much trouble to prepare?

★ If you don't like preparing them, perhaps you could eat them more often when you're out. Could you make healthier choices in restaurants? The healthiest menu options are usually the ones with fresh vegetables, salad or fruit – then you don't have to do the preparation.

★ How about preparing some fruit and veggies in advance, chopping up enough for a day and putting them in a plastic box?

- ★ Do you like frozen vegetables? They're convenient and they're better than no vegetables at all.
- ★ Could you put fruit on your breakfast cereal?

Do you really not like fruit and vegetables?

- ★ Sorry, but that's impossible – there are so many different tastes and textures that you couldn't possibly dislike *all* of them.
- ★ If you don't like the taste of the fruit or vegetables you're familiar with, could you try some different ones until you find ones you do like?
- ★ If it's the texture, stop and think about which fruit and vegetables have textures you don't like: what's putting you off? Are they too mushy? Or too juicy? Or too hard? Too many bits that get in your teeth? Pause now to think about some options that you're pretty sure would have completely different textures and add them to your ongoing shopping list in the Diary. You did start one, didn't you?
- ★ If it's vegetables that bother you more than fruit, do you eat them cooked or raw? How about eating them raw if you don't like them cooked? And what about experimenting with some different ways of cooking them? Steaming or roasting them often gives them more flavour.

A STRATEGY FOR CHANGE

My friend Lisa would never eat fruit and I once asked her why.

'My mother used to put an apple in my lunchbox and it was always bruised by the time I got round to it.'

'Oranges?'

'Too many pips. Can't be bothered.'

'Bananas?'

'Yuck! Mashed banana. It's the only thing I remember being fed as a baby. Bananas are not grown-up food.'

It seemed like just about everything had some kind of childhood memory attached to it. Then I decided to get more exotic.

'Mangoes?'

'Don't know, never tried one.'

'Lychees?'

'They taste all right out of a tin. I've never had fresh ones.'

That gave me an idea. Perhaps if Lisa tried some fruit she *hadn't* eaten as a child, she could make a fresh start on getting her daily vitamins. Next time she came round I put a plate of fresh fruit on the table instead of pudding.

By the end of the evening she admitted she was ready for a rethink. 'Mind you,' she said, 'it's a lot more effort than a Mars bar. But it's probably worth it.'

I've tried this idea on many people since then and it usually works. I still know a few people who will *only* eat strawberries, or peeled apples, or overripe bananas and absolutely nothing else that grows on a tree. But 99.9 per cent of people will reluctantly admit that maybe, just maybe, they might be ready to be more adventurous.

Carbohydrates

We've already talked about sugar, which is a simple carbohydrate. The more complex carbohydrates, contained in grains and many vegetables, are much better for you – but unfortunately it's the simple ones, the sugars in sweets, biscuits and soft drinks, that are a lot more tempting to most people.

HIGH-QUALITY STODGE

Eating complex carbohydrates, which are low-fat and high-volume foods, is probably the best way to change your body shape for the better. Complex carbohydrates include wholemeal bread, cereals, grains and potatoes (and other fruit and vegetables as well). They release energy over long periods and stop you feeling hungry. They taste starchy and are high in nutritional value unless they've been processed or refined. But the really great thing about them is that up to 25 per cent of their calorific content can be burnt up during digestion.

Carbohydrates should provide about 50 per cent of our daily diet and it's a good idea to include at least one complex carbohydrate with each meal. Wherever you can, choose an unprocessed whole grain, such as brown rice, or products that are made with unrefined flour and no added sugars or salt. These unprocessed foods are a good source of fibre and give you plenty of energy.

Processed foods, like white flour, white rice, normal pasta and white bread, have lost their tough seeds and fibres. Not only do these seeds and fibres help the gut deal with the food, they also contain some of the vitamins and minerals. Refined foods are much lower in both fibre and nutritional value.

BREAD, CEREALS AND GRAINS

These are the most well-known carbohydrates. Wherever you can, look for unrefined whole products like rice, bulgar wheat and couscous. Most only need boiling and are simple to prepare – but some take a little time. If you fancy something different, go to your local health food shop and try some of the more unusual grains like buckwheat, millet and spelt.[3]

But don't forget that lots of other fruits and vegetables, including beans and lentils, also provide good-quality complex carbohydrates.

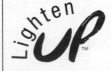 *If you're stuck for ideas, use some of the recipes at the back of this book or go and buy one of the hundreds of easy and appealing cookery books with imaginative recipes for preparing grains.*

Fat

WHY FAT MAKES YOU FAT

The human body has a really easy time converting the fat you eat into the fat you wear. It only takes 2.5 calories to turn 100 calories of the fat you've eaten into fat on your bum. But converting carbohydrate or protein into fat takes a lot more biochemical processing and a lot more energy. In fact, converting 100 calories of protein or carbohydrate into fat for storage can take up to 25 calories – ten times the number needed to process

3 There's a much bigger list in Chapter Seventeen.

---

the equivalent amount of fat. So even with the same calorie intake, a high-fat diet is more likely to lead to weight gain than a high-carbohydrate or high-protein diet. You shouldn't stop eating fat, we all need it, but you can make sure you eat only as much as you use. The fitter you are, the more efficient you will be at burning fat.

Fat is a valuable source of energy and protects against heat loss. It contains twice the calories (9 per gram) of either protein or carbohydrate. So if you plan to walk across the Antarctic, towing your own sledge, it should definitely be the main part of your diet.

But for sedentary non-Eskimos, fat is seen as something of an enemy, which is realistic. And about 60 per cent of fats are hidden in foods like cakes, chocolates, biscuits and crisps, which means we don't always realise how much we're eating. But once we cut down on, or cut out, these foods, our fat intake will be lowered quite substantially.

We need *some* fat in our diet because it contains vitamins A, D, E and K, which are essential for a healthy body. It also protects our vital organs, it's a valuable source of energy and provides flavouring for many foods. And we need fat to burn fat.

 How many of these guidelines do you follow?

1 Using skimmed or low-fat milk, non-fat or low-fat yoghurt.
2 Cutting down or cutting out cakes, chocolates, sweets and crisps.
3 Eating meat in modest portions, choosing lean cuts and limiting the use of processed meat.
4 Using olive oil when you're cooking, instead of saturated fat.
5 Eating plenty of fruit and vegetables. They are a good supply of fibre, vitamins and minerals, as well as being low in fat and having no cholesterol.
6 Eating wholegrain bread.
7 Trimming off the fat and removing the skin before you cook meat.
8 Using non-stick pans and olive oil for frying.

9 Substituting low-fat or non-fat plain yoghurt for sour cream or mayonnaise.
10 Grilling or baking meat instead of frying it.
11 Reading the labels on all pre-prepared food from biscuits to pizza.
12 Eating more fish – it's low in saturated fat, cholesterol and calories, and it's a good source of protein, B vitamins and zinc.

If you follow less than six of those on a regular basis, how many more of them could you start doing from today? Make a note of this in your Diary.

CUTTING BACK

As you already know from last week, sugar doesn't add much to our diet. Fat, on the other hand, is essential – though many people eat more of it than they need.

Cutting back on both sugar and fat will give you a much healthier diet; one that will help you to be slimmer, fitter and healthier, as well as reducing the risk of many illnesses and longer-term physical malfunctions and discomforts.

Thirty years ago obesity was less common. People ate more than they do now, but they also took more exercise. And their food was more natural, with a higher proportion of fruit and vegetables and less pre-packed, chemically created products. The amount of fat and sugar in most people's diet was also considerably lower than it is now.

SUGAR AND FAT TOGETHER

When you eat a bar of chocolate or a triple-layer fudge cake, there is a sudden explosion of pleasure on your taste buds, but it's short-lived. Your fat cells are immediately filled and your blood vessels are left coated and clogged. The sugar hit also puts a great strain on your regulatory system because the sugar is absorbed so quickly into the bloodstream. It's like doing something selfish which causes pain to a friend. You upset them and then leave them alone to sort out all the bad feelings. When you eat sugar and fat together your body is left with a lot of damage to repair – the result of your craving for instant pleasure.

★ Fat and sugar mixes are highly refined and (as in shop-bought cakes) often loaded with chemicals.
★ This combination doesn't satisfy hunger so you don't know when you've had enough.
★ You can eat a lot of calories in this form without feeling full, which is why people often say they haven't eaten much – they don't think they have!
★ The fat and sugar combination activates huge amounts of digestive enzymes, which make short work of your snack and send messages to the brain requesting more food. This is why most people can't eat just one chocolate – you may find that after a fat and sugar snack you feel even hungrier than you did before.

If you put the wrong octane petrol in your car it won't run very well and you'll be causing long-term damage. If you try to run your body on cream buns and biscuits you're putting it under tremendous strain as you pile on the pounds. Your body's going to be less reliable, its performance will suffer and, if it breaks down completely, you can't replace it.

FASTER FAT

Technological advances have increased the quality and range of convenience meals that are now available. We can get fat faster than ever before and with minimal expenditure of energy. We don't even have to go and collect our takeaways, now that home delivery is so widespread. Vacuum-packed or frozen, pre-cooked, microwaveable, meal-type foods are readily available just about everywhere. Who wants simple bread, cheese and an apple for supper when they can pick up three courses from the corner shop on their way home from the station? In fact, there are some things we just don't bother to prepare at home any more: when did you last make a hamburger, assuming mad cows haven't put you off the idea altogether? If you're working long hours, or you're trying to run a home, raise a family and study for your degree at the same time, convenience foods can be very appealing.

However, though life may be too short to stuff a mushroom, as Shirley Conran once said, at least you'd know what you were stuffing the mushroom with. According to the study on sugar consumption we mentioned earlier [4] almost every convenience food contains a much higher proportion of sugar than a similar recipe made at home. The reason for this is that it's much more cost-effective to make something palatable by adding sugar (and salt), rather than by using more of the expensive fresh ingredients. Regardless of whether or not they're masquerading as complete meals, these easy meals are rarely an adequate source of vegetables or complex carbohydrates.

Fast-food restaurants and takeaways are becoming more and more popular, especially with children. There's more variety and food quality is better now than it was ten years ago. But they still don't measure up well nutritionally. A typical cheeseburger and chips with apple pie and a large Coke contains between 1100 and 1200 calories. And a lot of those calories come from saturated fats and sugar. The drink alone (besides colouring, chemicals and caffeine) contains around seven teaspoons of sugar. The main reason our fat intake is up by 50 per cent is largely due to the fast-food revolution. We're overfed and undernourished because it's easy to eat packaged food full of fats that have been heated and hydrogenated so our bodies don't know how to deal with them.

But sadly, although the typical takeaway is high in saturated fat, salt and sugar, and low in fibre, there are still more people snacking on fries than on fruit.

CONVENIENCE FOODS

So next time you're tempted to go for a takeaway or a ready meal, stop and ask yourself if it's really worth it:

★ What are you going to do with the time you save on preparing that meal? Is it time worth saving? Or could you have just as much fun in the kitchen? If you really need to save that time, ask how much longer it would take you to make

4 Dr William Grant, NASA, February, 1999.

yourself a healthy sandwich, wash some salad, open a tin of tuna, or peel a banana. A proper meal doesn't necessarily have to be cooked.

★ How about making your own fast food ? There are a number of really rapid-to-prepare recipes that taste a lot better than anything you can buy. I've included some of them at the end of this book.

And if you really can't persuade yourself out of that convenience food:

★ Why not add an extra portion of vegetables, or a salad? You might possibly even add an easy complex carbohydrate such as brown rice or a wholemeal bread roll.

★ When you eat at a junk-food restaurant, skip the melted cheese and mayonnaise.

★ Some fast-food places offer slightly healthier alternatives now – including salad bars. Look out for them.

★ Always run Think Before You Eat and check out how that food is going to make you feel after you've eaten it.

 When you went shopping, did you plan your meals for the next week? If not, write down at least one simple meal or snack you could prepare for each day of this week in place of convenience food. Put them in your Diary and tick each one off when you prepare it.

Water

DRINK LOTS OF WATER

★ Water is an essential part of our bodily needs, second only to oxygen. It makes up approximately 55–65 per cent of an adult's body weight and approximately 75 per cent of a child's.

★ Two litres are lost on average every 24 hours. This loss rises dramatically during exercise, depending on the duration and intensity of the exercise, your level of hydration before you start and the air temperature.

★ Water loss accounts for the weight loss you measure immediately after exercise.

★ It's used by the body to aid temperature control. In situations where people sweat excessively, such as hot weather, exercise or illness, it's important to drink a lot more of it.

★ Water is essential to digestion and elimination. As a cleanser it's crucial in allowing the kidneys to flush out toxins more effectively. Constant replenishment is vital to feeling and looking good.

★ It acts as a lubricant in the joints and between internal organs, keeping cells moist and allowing the passage of all manner of internal substances between cells and blood vessels.

Drink two to three litres a day, preferably pure. Although everything you drink is water based – orange juice, squash, Coke, coffee and tea – the more things that are added to it, the longer it will take to extract the vital water. So if your favourite drinks are full of E numbers (chemicals) or caffeine (some soft drinks contain both) they won't be as beneficial to your system. Also, most soft drinks are full of sugar – between seven and fifteen spoonfuls!

Remember that Coca-Cola and similar drinks, together with coffee and tea, are diuretics, which means they actually dehydrate you by making you secrete more fluid than you take in. That is another reason some people feel below par a lot of the time: they're simply dehydrated.

The bottom line is that water in its purest form is how the body likes it.

 How many of these habits do you already have? Make a note in your Diary to start doing the others.

★ Drink a glass of water in the morning before breakfast.

★ Drink water whenever you drink alcohol, tea or coffee.

★ In colder weather it's sometimes tempting to drink more coffee and tea than water. Cold water can be very chilling on a cold day – but you could always drink warmer water in colder weather.

★ Take water with you on long car journeys or to work.

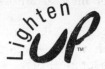

Drink little and often. Don't force yourself to drink pints at a time if you don't want to. A lot of people go for hours without a drink and then force themselves to down half a litre in one go, just to make up for it. You should never feel bloated and waterlogged. Just keep sipping and watch out for thirst signals. You'll be surprised at how much water your body asks you for once you start to listen to it.

HOW TO BE A BREATHARIAN

And now it's time to take a breather.

A year or so ago there was a lot of publicity about a group of people calling themselves Breatharians. These people apparently believed it was possible to get all the nutrients a human being needs from the air and that eating was unnecessary. I heard that the leader of the cult was caught ordering a vegetarian meal on a transatlantic flight and as far as I know they haven't had much airtime since then. Of course, plenty of meat eaters would maintain that vegetarian meals aren't real food – so perhaps that was her excuse.

I can't vouch for the truth of any of that. But I have met a lot of people who have joined the Breatharian cult under another name – anorexia. The glut of food in the Western world and the fashion for extreme thinness have put us in a terrible dilemma. To many people food is as desirable and dangerous as heroin. They can't live with it and they can't live without it.

BREATHING AS A MEAL SUBSTITUTE

In spite of what the Breatharians believe, you can't live on air, whether it's fresh, polluted or oxygen-enriched. But they do have a point. It could be very beneficial to a lot of overweight (and overstressed) people if they substituted some of their non-necessary meals or snacks with deep breathing and relaxation exercises.

BREATHING THROUGH YOUR NOSE

Many overweight people seem to be quite shallow breathers for some reason and if you think that might apply to you there is something you can do about it. Deep breathing and relaxation techniques are a very important part of the Lighten Up programme:

★ Do you breathe through your mouth? Well, stop it and start breathing through your nose. Your nose was designed for breathing and filtering air, and your mouth wasn't. Breathing straight into your mouth sends an emergency signal to your body. Most people breathe quickly through their mouths when they panic. If you breathe through your mouth a lot, it may be making your whole body tight and tense, and perhaps even encouraging your body to hold on to its fat stores.

★ Deeper breathing provides your body with more oxygen and the more oxygen you take in the more fat you can burn. And there's a bonus with deep breathing – it helps you relax and feel good.

★ Controlling your breathing also helps you take control of your emotional state, so you can protect yourself against those moments of vulnerability when you might resort to overeating.

★ It also has a direct physical benefit: you can digest your food more easily if your muscles are relaxed. Most people know this – you're much more likely to get indigestion if you eat when your stomach's clenched, which is hardly surprising when you think how much that's likely to restrict all your digestive organs.

★ Deeper breathing will help you to exercise more effectively.

 JUST BREATHING

Put one hand on your chest and one on your stomach. Take a deep, gentle breath. Which hand moves the most? It should be your stomach but it's more likely to be your chest.

Practise breathing in and feeling your stomach rise as your lungs fill with air. As you breathe out again, feel your stomach sinking back towards your spine.

BREATHING AWAY STRESS

★ Stand rigidly upright with your hands by your side and fists clenched.

★ Tense all your muscles and slowly breathe in as you rise up on to your toes.

★ Hold the breath for a count of three, shoulders hunched, muscles contracted. Find a point ahead of you to stare at and this will help you keep your balance.

★ As you start to breathe out, slowly relax all your muscles from your neck to your toes, lowering your feet flat on to the floor. You should be in the orang-utan position, with droopy hands, sloping shoulders and bent knees.

★ Do this five times.

WALKING AND BREATHING: FOUR MINUTES

Don't laugh. Not everybody can do this.

★ Walk at a steady pace, wait until you have got into your stride.

★ Breathe in deeply for a couple of paces.

★ Hold that breath for a couple of paces.

★ Breathe out for two paces.

★ Relax as you breathe and keep doing this for as long as you feel comfortable.

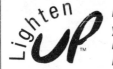

Next time you feel the urge to eat, check where you are on the Hunger Scale. If you're registering less than 6, try some deep breathing instead.

It's a good idea to practise deeper breathing in your daily life rather than just doing it as a special occasional exercise. Breathe more deeply when you're just chatting, travelling or watching TV; breathe deeply as you exercise and especially when you happen to be in a stressful situation.

LOOKING FOR A GOOD TIME

DO THIS NOW At this point in the Lighten Up programme you're probably becoming more aware of your eating patterns and the reasons you may be eating when you aren't hungry. A quick fix of pleasure is one of the main reasons for eating apart from hunger and, of course, eating should be a great source of pleasure – but *only* when you're hungry.

So where else, apart from food, can you get the rest of your daily pleasure quota? Where do you get it from right now?

Cooking food
Dancing
Drinking alcohol
Eating chocolate
Eating takeaways
Exercising
Going to parties
Going to the cinema
Listening to music
Looking after children
Looking good
Netsurfing
Playing football
Reading novels
Shopping
Smoking
Spending time with friends
Taking drugs
Taking long walks
Watching films
Watching football
Watching TV

....

....

....

Be honest, write *everything* down. The next job is sorting out the acceptable displacement activities from the ones that are just as bad for you as overeating. A lot of people have a cigarette instead of a biscuit with their coffee. It serves the same purpose – it distracts them from being unhappy – and they don't gain weight. But the health risks are high.[5]

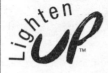 Ask yourself, 'What are the long-term effects of my favourite activities?' Don't choose an eating substitute that's going to give you yet another problem to deal with.

DISPLACEMENT ACTIVITIES

DO SOMETHING ELSE

You can develop a whole repertoire of alternatives to food – and just think how interesting your life could become once you start getting creative with this particular strategy. For example, you might look for activities that will

★   meet some of your un-hungry needs more directly. If it's not food your body's after, perhaps you could figure out what you really want and have that instead – like a snooze or a chat or just a break from routine;
★   make you feel good (exercise and deep breathing).

Don't leave yourself vulnerable, lonely or uncomforted. If you are triggered to eat for any other reason than hunger, ask yourself:

5 According to a National Audit Office report in November 1999, the NHS was spending £1.73 billion a year on treating overweight people who suffered from conditions directly linked to their weight, such as heart disease, strokes, diabetes and even cancer. This exceeded the £1.5 billion spent on diseases related to smoking.

★ What do I really want?
★ What can I do (other than eating) to make myself feel good?

Finding something different that hits the right spot may take a little time. And doing it might meet with some resistance at first – in your own mind and in other people's. We tend to be creatures of habit and comfort. When we find something that makes us feel better, we usually stop looking for other alternatives, even if our chosen method (like eating) has negative side-effects. It's better to keep looking.

Look past the initial resistance, past the first hurdles, and see what your new patterns will do for you in future. Keep your eye on this and there's a good chance you'll start to enjoy doing things differently.

When an emotion creeps over you that used to trigger you to eat you'll find yourself doing something else instead. The more often you repeat your new behaviour, the easier it will become and eventually you'll find your new habit has a stronger pull on you than eating used to have.

 Here are some ideas. Have a look through them and tick the ones you do already. Then put a star against the ones you are going to do this week. Break the tyranny of your eating triggers by learning to recognise them and then reprogramming yourself to react to them differently.

Arrange to play tennis
Book a holiday
Buy a really nice wine and share it
Buy a relaxation tape
Buy a tape or CD
Buy fancy underwear
Buy flowers for yourself or someone else
Catch up on some sewing
Check your credit card bills
Clean all your shoes

Clean your car or your bike
Clear out a cupboard
Design your ideal bedroom
Design your ideal house
Do a jigsaw
Do the ironing
Do your breathing exercises
Do your tax return
Draw or paint a picture
Feed some ducks
Fit in a Feel Good Fitness session
Get online and surf the net
Give someone else a massage
Go fishing
Go for a walk
Go skating
Go swimming
Go to a football game
Go to a museum
Go to an aerobics or stretch class
Have a facial
Have a massage
Have a nap
Introduce yourself to a neighbour
Invite friends to play cards
Join a political party
Listen to live music
Make a list of everything you want to do next year
Meditate
Mend something
Pet a cat or dog
Phone a friend
Pick fresh fruit
Picnic
Plan a holiday
Plan a party
Plan an outing on your next free day
Plant something

Play solitaire
Polish some silver or brass
Prepare to decorate a room
Read a book
Rearrange the furniture
Rewrite your address book
Ride a bike
See a movie
Send a card
Set up a murder evening
Set yourself up with a date
Sort out your wardrobe
Start a new evening class
Start learning a language
Stick some photos in an album
Take a Fat-Burning Pill
Take music lessons
Take some children on an outing
Take up knitting
Throw out some jumble
Tidy up your tights
Try a new computer program
Visit a bird sanctuary or aquarium
Visit another town
Visit the library
Volunteer for a charity
Wash the curtains
Wash the leaves on your plants
Watch the sunset
Window shop
Write a letter

Now add two more of your own ideas:

1 ....

2 ....

Remember the theory that it takes 20 to 30 times for a new pattern or behaviour to become automatic? Don't give up too soon.

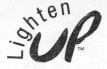

If you end up eating the Danish pastry instead of sorting out your wardrobe , forget about it. It's done. Do it differently next time. But don't prolong the agony when you've had a little lapse – you're only reinforcing your fat image when you do that.

THE LIGHTEN UP DIARY

New Notes:

★ Which of the guidelines for cutting down on fat are you going to follow? Write them down.

★ How much water are you drinking? If you're not drinking enough, make a note of a couple of ways you could increase your water consumption.

★ Make a note every time you leave food on your plate. Maybe you leave some already, but if it's something you *never* do, it's very important. For some of us it's an ingrained habit, reinforced by commands we were given long before we could understand them logically. Nobody could possibly ever get the right amount on their plate every time. If you never leave anything, there must be times when you're eating more than you're hungry for.

Carry On:

★ filling in the Food Profile, remembering to include everything you drink;

★ making a note of:
  - where you are on the Hunger Scale whenever you eat;
  - any remaining eating patterns that you would still like to get rid of;
  - every time you use Think Before You Eat – how fast can you do this now and how accurate are the results?
  - any lapses you have and whether the success formula in Week Four helped you to cope.

CHALLENGES

★ Add a new displacement activity to your food-coping strategies. Which one are you going to choose? Write it down now.

★ Try out a new form of carbohydrate, a new kind of fruit and a different vegetable this week. Choose things you've never eaten before and experiment with some new recipes.

★ Make sure you do at least three Feel Good Fitness sessions and add a fourth one if you would like to.

★ Don't forget you're going to replace at least one fast-food meal with a simple, home-prepared snack this week. What are you going to make? Write it down.

★ Continue to separate eating from your other activities whenever you can. Slow it down and savour it.

★ Get rid of another unwanted eating pattern (if you have any left).

CHECKLIST FOR WEEK FIVE

Weekly checklist

Which eating pattern are you going to eliminate this week?
Write it here:

....

On which three days are you going to do your Feel Good Fitness
sessions? Write them here:

Feel Good Fitness session 1: ....

Feel Good Fitness session 2: ....

Feel Good Fitness session 3: ....

And one for luck? ....

	Day 1	Day 2	Day 3	Day 4	Day 5	Day 6	Day 7
Daily checklist							
The Movie: polishing up your self-motivation	☐	☐	☐	☐	☐	☐	☐
Breathing exercises	☐	☐	☐	☐	☐	☐	☐
First Fat Burning Pill	☐	☐	☐	☐	☐	☐	☐
Second Fat Burning Pill	☐	☐	☐	☐	☐	☐	☐
First Affirmation session	☐	☐	☐	☐	☐	☐	☐
Second Affirmation session	☐	☐	☐	☐	☐	☐	☐
Congratulating yourself on an achievement before you go to sleep at night	☐	☐	☐	☐	☐	☐	☐
The Lighten Up Diary	☐	☐	☐	☐	☐	☐	☐

My goal for the rest of the programme is:

....

....

CHAPTER FOURTEEN

WEEK SIX
OF THE
EIGHT-WEEK
COURSE

HOW ARE YOU DOING?

You're going to start noticing changes. As you increase the activity in your daily routine, you'll see a knock-on effect on your lifestyle and energy levels. Be prepared to congratulate yourself when these positive things start happening.

Now that you are getting into the routine of the Lighten Up Diary you may be finding yourself increasingly intrigued by some of the things you're learning about yourself. Things like the feelings you associate with what and when you eat, and how much better you're starting to feel about eating as you take time to enjoy your food.

Some changes take a little longer than others. Sometimes it's the simplest things that seem the hardest. Leaving food on your plate, for example, is almost impossible for some of us. Some people really can't tell the difference between their bodies and the kitchen bin. And lots of us hear old messages being replayed when we try to put a few potatoes on the compost heap, or give some of the fatty bits of meat to the dog.

In order to change, we have to challenge the beliefs we still live by, but which no longer work for us. And we are in a stronger position to stand up to our past and to our old beliefs if we're feeling strong and positive about ourselves and convinced of our own ability to succeed.

LAST WEEK'S LIGHTEN UP DIARY AND CHALLENGES

★ Did you enjoy running the Movie? If you use this kind of visualisation regularly, the future you want will be so clear that you will soon find it much easier to motivate yourself to make changes. Get into the habit of visualising what you want to happen and saying your everyday affirmations to yourself as you use your imagination. This is a powerful and convincing technique for helping yourself to reach your goals.

★ How are you getting on with your Fat Jar? Is the Borg Scale helping you to do your Feel Good Fitness at the right level? And how many Feel Good Fitness sessions did you manage to do? Are you keeping up to three a week – or are you up to four sessions now? Are you paying attention to your breathing when you exercise?

★ Are you noticing any change in the balance of your Food Profile? If you were missing out on some of your fresh fruit and veggies before, is that section filling up now? Are you enjoying the difference in your diet?

★ Do you eat some of your meals slowly and without doing anything else at the same time?

★ Did you manage to substitute a real meal for a pre-prepared or takeaway at least once? And are you preparing food differently in any way – so as to include less fat, for example?

★ How much water did you drink last week? If you're drinking more water than you did before, does that mean that you're drinking less of other things? Or about the same?

★ Are you still consciously using the Hunger Scale and Think Before You Eat? Or is it all down to intuition now? These two processes will eventually become so instinctive, you may stop noticing yourself running them. Be patient if you aren't there yet. Just keep reminding yourself to do them and one day you will suddenly discover that you're doing it automatically.

★ What did you eat this week that you never ate before? A new fruit or vegetable? A different type of carbohydrate? Did you like it? Do you plan to experiment some more?

★ How effective are the displacement activities? Did you find at least one that could distract you from a habitual snacking pattern? Did you use it to get rid of one of your remaining eating patterns? If not, what *did* you do? Did it work?

★ Have you been using the deep-breathing exercises? Do you feel calmer when you do some deep breathing? And does that help you *not* to bury your feelings under food?

★ How many lapses did you have last week? And how did you deal with them?

★ Are you giving yourself a regular pat on the back whenever you deserve it – as well as calling your daily successes to mind before you fall asleep at night?

Are You Ready?

Until now you've probably been doing this on your own or with a sympathetic friend. This week we're encouraging you to take some of your new strategies out for a test drive. Maybe you've already been using Think Before You Eat and the Hunger Scale in restaurants. Or putting your knife and fork down between bites. Or turning down an invitation for a beer and going for a walk instead.

But if you've been keeping these good ideas to yourself until now it's time to put yourself in the front line. Get together with some friends who still have the lifestyle and eating habits you're leaving behind. See if they can talk you back into the error of your old ways.

If you can stand up to the sabotage test you're doing well.

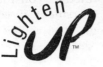

WEEK SIX

This week we'll be looking at the reasons why you adopted a lifestyle that led to you being overweight. It's about awareness of what you do and why you do it, and there will be a lot of leeway to do your own thinking round the subject. Doing your own thinking is a very useful tool for building a slimmer future – or any kind of future you want.

★ The Food Profile: this week it's protein, dairy products, nuts and seeds that come under the spotlight.
★ Alcohol.
★ Healthy Cooking.
★ Health Food for the Mind: being aware of what you do, so you can do things differently, and giving yourself support and encouragement to change.
★ Sabotage: dealing with pressure from other people.
★ Rewrite the Rules: doing things differently.
★ Stress: how to cope without resorting to overeating.
★ Putting More Effort into Relaxation: preparing to learn more about coping with stress.
★ Listen to Your Body: learning to trust your intuition.

THE FOOD PROFILE

Our final look at the Food Profile is a review of proteins, dairy products, nuts and seeds and, as I've mentioned before, you'll find more detailed information about food groups and nutrition in Chapter Seventeen if you're interested.

Once again we must emphasise that the Food Profile isn't a set of rules. Now you know how important it is for your health and slimness to eat a fresh, varied diet, you'll always be aware of what you're eating on a daily basis. But it's flexible – if you're travelling, or your exercise levels are higher or lower, or you're pregnant, or elderly, or you have some other special requirement – be prepared to adapt.

You should also bear in mind that the scientific study of nutrition is still quite new. Discoveries are being made all the time about the effects on our bodies of the food we eat, and the Lighten Up panel of experts will be on hand to keep you updated with current information. If you want to be in on the latest news, check our website (www.lightenup.co.uk), or call our office (see page 419) and make sure you get a copy of the *Lighten Update*, our regular newsletter.

Protein

Every cell in the body needs protein. We need it to grow and repair everything from muscles and bones to hair and finger-nails. Ideally you should get your protein from several different sources (the varied diet again) but there's no point in eating too much at a time because our bodies can't store it.

Protein is actually made up of amino acids and the foods that contain all the acids are called complete proteins. These are mostly animal in origin: meat, poultry, eggs and fish. Soya beans (and tofu which is made from soya beans) are the only non-animal foods that are complete proteins.

Vegetables that contain some but not all of the amino acids are called incomplete proteins and if we mix them together in the right combinations our bodies can make up the missing amino acids.

HERBIVORE OR CARNIVORE?

It's possible to be a very healthy vegetarian. But because veg-etable proteins are incomplete (apart from soya), vegetarians, and especially vegans and fruitarians, need to take more care over what they eat. If you restrict your diet – whether it's because you're vegetarian or simply because there's a type of food you don't like – take expert advice and make sure you're getting all the essential nutrients.

Vegetable sources of protein

Even if you're not a vegetarian, it's still a good idea to include some vegetarian sources of protein in your diet as red meat is particularly high in fat and has been linked to heart disease. Fortunately there are plenty of good-quality protein sources in cereals (wheat, oats, rice and bread), in pulses (peas, beans and lentils) and in nuts, seeds and potatoes. Beans, including soya, tofu and lentils, are particularly good. If you eat them with a grain such as rice or bread (beans on toast or lentil dhal with rice, for example) – you'll be getting all the proteins you need. Vegetable proteins also contain both soluble and insoluble fibre, which is great for your health in other ways, as we'll mention later.

Apart from the sweetened baked beans which grace the full English breakfast, many people never eat pulses at all. If you're one of the majority who doesn't think they're real food, give them a try. Buy some chick peas, broad beans, black-eyed beans, mung beans, green and red lentils, red kidney beans or borlotti beans and experiment with some of the recipes at the end of the book.

And if you're a carnivore . . .
★ Choose lean meat, fish and poultry without skin.
★ Prepare meat in low fat ways by trimming it and not frying it.
★ Increase the proportion of fish and chicken in your diet rather than red meat and dairy food.

Dairy products, nuts and seeds

These food groups get a special mention here, because they're rich in many key nutrients.

DAIRY FOODS

Dairy foods are a good source of protein and carbohydrate but they also contain lots of fat and cholesterol. Go for the foods with a lower fat content if you can, otherwise you may use up all your daily fat servings in one go.

★ Use skimmed or semi-skimmed milk.
★ Eat low-fat cheese.
★ Substitute live yoghurt for ice-cream, milkshakes and sweetened yoghurt.
★ Stick to only one egg yolk in a serving.

It is best to spread out your servings of dairy foods rather than eating them all in one sitting. And watch out for the hidden sugars in some dairy products, as well as the fats.

NUTS AND SEEDS

Nuts and seeds are high in calories, but they're not empty calories by any means. They're another underrated and neglected source of protein, vitamins and essential fatty acids. Their reputation has suffered since they became a cocktail snack and a lot of people still won't eat them because they think they're too fattening. Well, they are fattening, but they're also very high in nutritional value so as long as you eat them when you're physically hungry, they're also good for you. And they taste great.

Seeds and nuts make delicious healthy snacks. And they're very easy to add to meals. Pumpkin, sesame and sunflower seeds taste wonderful on a whole range of vegetable dishes and salads. Roasted ones tend to be acidic and heavily salted, so it's best to eat them fresh. All nuts contain useful nutrients but some are higher in saturated fat than others. If you'd like to know which ones are best to eat, take a look at the list in Chapter Seventeen.

Don't eat them if you have a nut allergy.

ALCOHOL

By now you should be clear on the need to cut down or cut out refined sugar. However, there's another equally harmful substance that many people are drawn to because it makes them feel even better than sugar. It has other attractions, too: it's very socially acceptable and it can be addictive.

Alcohol is a drug, but it's also the highest-calorie quick fix for stress, apart from overeating. It's fast becoming our third major health hazard in the UK after heart disease and cancer. There are 70 calories in a glass of wine, it doesn't add anything to your diet nutritionally and it can even cause vitamin deficiencies. Like sugar, it's absorbed into the bloodstream very quickly. Drinking alcohol can seriously harm your health and it only takes around four units a day, over a period of time, to cause liver damage in an average-size person.

Another problem with alcohol is that it stops you noticing how much you're eating. A study in the Netherlands found that drinking before and during meals made people eat more quickly and scoff bigger portions. It can remove your inhibitions and encourage you to eat more.

 Ask yourself 'Why do I drink?' and come up with at least ten answers. Either write these down here or in the Diary.

★ ....

★ ....

★ ....

★ ....

★ ....

★ ....

★ ....

★ ....

★ ....

★ ....

There's only one good reason for drinking alcohol and that's enjoyment, which means taking it slowly and savouring every sip. Look at the other reasons you came up with and ask yourself if any of them is more important to you than staying slim and healthy.

DRINKING RULES

★ Drink in moderation.
★ Drink water with alcohol and don't drink on an empty stomach.
★ Drink slowly and don't use it to wash down your food.
★ Never use it to quench thirst. It's a diuretic.

- ★ If you're drinking spirits, ask yourself if you might substitute wine or beer, which have a lower alcohol content.
- ★ Be aware of how alcohol is making you feel and how much you've drunk.
- ★ Drink at your own pace, unless it's faster than everybody else's.
- ★ The fewer chemicals in your chosen drink, the less harm it will do you. Read the labels.
- ★ If you drink spirits at home, think small pub measures.
- ★ Spend more on buying high quality and drink less of it.

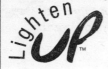 *Using alcohol as a quick fix is a really bad idea. You will feel temporarily relaxed, but, like overeating, drinking alcohol leaves your body with damage to repair.*

HEALTHY COOKING

Preparing your own fresh food – even if it's just peeling your own banana or making yourself a sandwich – is generally a healthier option than buying something ready prepared. Cooking for yourself (and your friends) is one of the things we suggest you do more often.

 Go through this list and put a cross against everything you already do (we mentioned some of these ideas in Week Five). Then put a tick against all the new ideas you will try out this week. Write these down in your Diary.

- ★ Eat plenty of vegetables.
- ★ Grill rather than fry.
- ★ Choose white meat and fish in preference to red meat.
- ★ Reduce the amount of added sugar.
- ★ Reduce the amount of added cream and high-fat cheese.
- ★ Trim the fat and the skin from meat.

- ★ Reduce the amount of oil you use in cooking and dressings.
- ★ Roast vegetables – you don't really need fat if you use a non-stick or well-seasoned roasting tin.
- ★ Roast meat and let the fat drain.
- ★ Reduce the amount of added salt.
- ★ Steam vegetables.
- ★ Remove the fat from the meat juice before making gravy.
- ★ Check the recipes at the back of the book for ideas.
- ★ Find tastes you love. If you're forcing yourself to eat beetroot because it's supposed to be good for you and you hate it, eat something else.

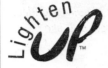 *As you get more relaxed about eating, you may find yourself tasting and enjoying foods that would never have crossed your mind or passed your lips before.*

HEALTH FOOD FOR THE MIND

We all know that we are what we eat. A fresh, healthy, balanced diet is a necessary stage on the journey to becoming slimmer and living a long life full of vitality and energy. We've been eating when we aren't physically hungry and, to make matters worse, we've been eating food that's often full of sugar, fat, chemicals, preservatives and additives, which can poison and confuse our bodies. Many dieters are so worried about calories and fat that they forget to look for all the other nasties. Before we take the first steps towards our slimmer, fitter selves, we need to start treating our bodies with more respect. So if we're prepared to be kinder to our bodies, shouldn't we think twice about the poison we constantly feed our minds as well?

Giving yourself a hard time is like systematically ingesting small doses of arsenic. There's no point in filling your mind with junk: 'I'm stupid . . . I can't do this . . . I'm fat . . . He won't like me . . .' Start listening to what you say to yourself and noticing how you treat yourself. This may feel strange at first, but persevere.

BE NICE TO YOURSELF

Our culture has taught us to be our own toughest critics. We are obsessed with problems. The most popular television programmes are soap operas, current affairs, news and disaster programmes. When people get together they talk about what's wrong with their lives: their house is too small, their salary is too low, their street is too noisy, their car is too old. It's more acceptable to talk about your problems than your triumphs (that's called boasting). Next time you walk down a busy street, take a look at how many people are smiling compared with those who look blank or miserable.

The most important thing to remember is that *you get what you focus on*. Focus on feeling good for no reason at all. Look for positive things in your life and you'll get more of them.

GET TO KNOW YOURSELF BETTER

 Answer these questions, either here or in your Diary. And then, for the rest of this week, pay special attention to your internal dialogue, listen to it, be curious about how you talk to yourself.

★ What sort of thing do you say when you talk to yourself?

....

★ Do you treat yourself as well as you treat your best friend? If not, what do you do differently?

....

★ What sort of messages do you give yourself? Can you give an example?

....

★ What do you talk to your friends about?

....

★ What do you read?

....

★ What do you watch?

....

Where is your attention – are you fascinated by problems, rather than solutions? If the evidence points this way, make sure you do some of the things on the following list:

★ If you start to give yourself a hard time, stop it.
★ If you hear a voice inside your head saying you're stupid, tell it to shut up.
★ When you talk to yourself, be polite, be gentle, be nice.
★ Give yourself encouragement.
★ Be kind to yourself.
★ Be your own best friend.

If you make a mistake, learn from it, laugh at it, leave it behind.

BEING YOUR OWN BEST FRIEND

It's an old saying that the first sign of madness is talking to yourself. Well, we all do it. But because we don't usually do it out loud, nobody notices, not even us. It's a good idea to become more aware of your internal dialogue.

As a sports trainer, I've seen a lot of people screaming verbal abuse at themselves (and sometimes at me) and it never makes the situation any better. Telling yourself you're an idiot is not going to improve your performance as a tennis player or a slimmer or anything else.

Many people who want to be slimmer discourage themselves in just the same way as these athletes. They want to look good and feel good but occasionally lapse into bad eating habits (unsurprisingly, as you can't change overnight) and then make things much worse by giving themselves a hard time: 'I should not have eaten that . . . I'm so stupid . . . I should have taken more exercise . . . I can't do it . . . I've got no will-power . . .'

That's just beating yourself up mentally and often this kind of social response is simply something we've learned from parents and teachers. The people who have successfully become slimmer have stopped battling with themselves. They've learned to be kind and accept themselves for who they are. They changed and so can you.

This is one of the most important principles of Lighten Up. If you want to be slimmer, the key is to be nicer to yourself. If you make yourself and your health and well-being your top priority, you have a high chance of success.

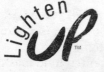 *Now that you're learning how to cope with self-sabotage and how to look after yourself, it's time to think up some strategies for coping with other people who try to bring you down (or build you up).*

SABOTAGE

What happens when you start to change but everyone around you stays the same? It makes no difference whether your friends and family have weight problems or not. Whether they are slim or overweight, they'll probably resist the changes in you to begin with. Don't panic. If the relationships are real and important, everything will be fine. If you lose someone you loved because you lost weight, the chances are the cracks were there already. It takes more than a few pounds of fat to wreck a relationship. Be brave, stick with your programme of change and, if it's right for you, the people who love you will love it in the end.

But be prepared. Sometimes people will try to make you eat. They may have lots of different reasons for doing this and you can have fun tailoring your avoidance strategy to their motivation. Just ask yourself what these people really mean when they hold out that plate of mini spring rolls and say, 'Oh, go on, you have to try these, they're yummy':

'I'm out to sabotage you.' People with weight problems hate it when they see someone else being strong-minded. You are responsible for your own health and happiness, but not for their state of mind. So say 'no thank you' and leave them to it.

'It's the only way I know to show I love you.' Some people can only show affection freely through offering food. This is particu-

larly true of older relatives and it requires a tactful response. After all, they may have lived through the war and known what it was like to eat bread and marrow jam for breakfast with no butter. If you see them often, tell them you have a food allergy and have to be careful what you eat. If you only see them every other Christmas either eat what they offer you graciously or tell them you got food poisoning yesterday and ask if you can take something home for when you're feeling better.

'It's the only way I know to ask you if you love me.' If you suspect that this is the real message, never mind the food; try just giving them a direct answer to the question. Like a hug.

'It's the only way I know to be sociable.' Very often food masks a social problem. Some people aren't very good at conversation and they find it's less embarrassing to feed you than to try to talk to you. If you're confronted with someone like this, distract them by talking to *them*, preferably about something other than eating. Always be sure to praise what they've prepared, even if you're not eating much of it. You can comment on how it looks and how long it must have taken – there's always something you can say without actually having to stuff yourself silly with it.

'I'm miserable, I'm going to overeat and I want company.' This is a dangerous one. You feel sorry for the person and you know how they feel. Try getting them to talk instead of eat. Or suggest an alternative solution like going to a movie together. If nothing will turn them from their self-destructive purpose, leave them to it. You may lose a friend – temporarily. But eating with them won't help.

SAS TACTICS

You can cope in difficult situations. Plan ahead and be prepared. Put together your own SAS (Sabotage Avoidance Strategies) plan. Here are a few that have been tried and tested:

 Try to predict the danger points of a social situation in advance. If you're not very assertive, don't be caught unawares. Rehearse some answers in case you find yourself in an eating-pressure situation.

Have you got something coming up that might tempt you to overeat? Write the date in your Diary and underneath devise three strategies you could use to make sure you don't pig out as usual. Here are some suggestions:

★ Eat only certain foods – go for the salad or sandwiches and leave the desserts.

★ Eat slowly. Start last and make it last.

★ Eat something before you go out; don't arrive at a special event starving.

★ When you're at a party, remember this is the only place and time when you can talk to this particular group of people – but you can eat peanuts at home whenever you want. Somebody in this room might be about to change your life, whether it's with a new idea, a job opportunity, a personal revelation, or a love affair.

★ Sit down to eat. Then you'll be more aware of starting and finishing.

★ Talk to other people about the food, praise the taste and style and presentation.

★ If it's a party, you could be the person who starts everybody dancing.

★ Offer to help in order to stay occupied.

★ Take what you want from the buffet table and then go and eat it somewhere else.

★ If you're drinking alcohol, don't let anyone top up your glass. Wait until you've finished one before starting another. That way, you'll know how much of a hangover you're entitled to.

★ When you've had enough just stop and explain you're full.

★ Remember, this is your life, your body, and you decide what goes in it.

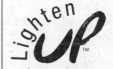

Think how good you will feel when you leave, knowing that you haven't overeaten.

REWRITE THE RULES

So you see, if social pressures to eat have brought you down in the past it doesn't matter. You're free to make up a whole new set of rules for dealing with them in future. Your circumstances might not change, the people around you might not change.

But you can change!

The secret of change is to do something differently from the way you were doing it before. Slimming is no exception. So if you've previously counted calories, cut out fat, carbohydrate, protein or puddings, and brought yourself to the edge of a heart attack by over-exercising, *you already know it doesn't work.*

Whether it's preparing and eating different foods, taking different kinds of exercise, or thinking of yourself in a different way, or indeed all those things, it's time to get used to change. And the first step is to give yourself a shot of pleasure to get you going. View yourself in a positive light. See yourself achieving your goal. Picture yourself becoming more active and enjoying it. Imagine what it would be like to eat a more varied and exciting diet.

Instead of cutting back and depriving yourself, how about experimenting with some different ways of cooking your food? You could make the process healthier by using less fat and sugar. Allow yourself to taste the food you cook, don't disguise it. Imagine you're training to become a gourmet, or a food taster for Fortnum & Mason. Tasting things bare is always an experience worth having. Sometimes it's like eating something for the first time when you find out what it's like without a coating of mustard or vinegar or soy sauce.

You'll discover what you really like and how food really tastes when you're hungry. You're starting from scratch and re-educating your taste buds. You'll find, when you begin eating this way, that you won't be able to eat as quickly as before and you'll feel fuller despite having eaten less than usual.

Always be sure that the food you eat satisfies you. Don't leave the table feeling hungry. That might feel like deprivation, and if you think you're being deprived you're likely to start resenting your change in eating habits.

STRESS

It's everywhere, it's an epidemic and if you haven't got it you obviously haven't lived.

Stress is credited with causing almost as much death and despair as war. It's been blamed for just about everything from migraine to cancer. The interesting thing is that it's not actually *out there* at all. It's just a feeling we mix for ourselves with our own personal chemicals.

THE TRUTH IS NOT OUT THERE

We blame it on social pressure, the new job, the new baby, the new relationship, or even the old job, the teenager and the divorce. But the truth is that what's stressful for one person will be exciting and challenging for another.

The pressures of a hectic social life make some people overeat. Other people overeat because they're alone and don't *have* a social life. But whether your overeating and poor self-image are caused by loneliness, other people or pressure of work doesn't matter. The end result is that you are overweight and even more unhappy than you were before. So it's time to identify your stress points and do something about them.

Stress isn't something you catch from someone else and it's not something other people do to you. There aren't even any universally stressful situations. If there were, there wouldn't be any surgeons, ambulance drivers and mercenary soldiers. There is no stress out there, not one bit. You've manufactured it yourself, tailored to your own personal tastes. You make the decisions about what you want to be stressful, whether it's losing your car keys, missing your train, overworking, boredom, or coping with a toddler. Hundreds of times a day we activate our personal stress response. Our brains start buzzing and breathing becomes faster as we get tense and tight. If this response becomes habitual we start to experience negative emotions like anger, sadness, low self-esteem and anxiety.

But we are also creatures of comfort and occasionally we need a break from all this stress and we look for a bit of pleasure to ease the pain. So we reach for the quick fixes: eating, smoking, drinking and whatever other chemicals are acceptable and affordable to us. The sadly predictable result is that any short-term relief is followed by a long-term intensification of the stress symptoms. Even more sadly, although stress itself doesn't actually exist, our reaction to it often causes very real health problems (like being overweight) and a poor quality of life (like feeling bad about ourselves and lacking confidence in relationships).

THE WORRY DUMP

 If anything on this page rings bells with you, if you know you're a worrier and that stress has you reaching for the comfort food, here's a neat little way of offloading it.

Spend two minutes, right now, writing a worry list. Time yourself and write everything down. You can do it in your Diary or on a piece of scrap paper. When you've done it, leave it there on the page and go away and do something that doesn't involve food. You can do this whenever things start getting on top of you – if you use a separate sheet of paper rather than putting it in the Diary you can even tear it up or burn it!

TWO WAYS OF DEALING WITH STRESS

Apart from doing a regular worry dump, there are two basic ways of dealing with stress: quick fixes and relaxation. If, like most people, you've always viewed the stress in your life as coming from outside yourself you're likely to look outside yourself for the cure – and that means a quick fix.

Quick fixes come in many forms – all of them bad for you. You may not think that a KitKat or a glass of wine can be compared with a line of cocaine, but if you're taking something to cover up feelings you can't cope with you're on the wrong tack whatever it is. It doesn't matter whether it's sex or popcorn – if you're using it just to ease the pain it may have painful side effects. The only good reason for eating is hunger and the only good reason to drink alcohol is for pleasure – not for escape.

Many people have very low expectations. They don't expect to feel good, they just hope to feel better – or make their unhappiness bearable for a while. This is true even of hard-drug users.

The first few hits may be ecstasy, but in the end most addicts are taking their drug just to survive – the first blissful experience has long since gone. They're only getting by, like the rest of us. But they made the mistake of thinking there was an easy way out.

I'm not saying you should *never* take any kind of drugs. Human beings have been artificially adjusting their brains for thousands of years. And some of the methods are so mild and well regulated by society that they don't have a terribly scary downside. There are times when a cup of tea or a glass of wine have far more benefits than disadvantages. And sometimes a chemical imbalance in the body needs a prescription from your doctor to sort it out. But before you reach for the bottle or the packet, make sure you weigh the short-term benefits against the long-term disadvantages.

Think past the immediate relief to the long-term result – what happens when the painkillers wear off? Will you feel as bad as you did before? Or worse? You can sit down in front of the TV with a pizza and a few beers and lose yourself in the problems of *EastEnders*. But when it's over you'll find your negative feelings haven't gone away – in fact, they've probably increased. Trying to solve your problems with a quick fix is like sweeping a huge pile of dust under the carpet. You might be able to pretend it isn't there for a while but it isn't going to go away. And sooner or later you're going to trip over the bump in the carpet and then you've got a whole other problem to add to your collection.

Quick Fixes

★ *Alcohol.* A depressant. Expensive, smelly, damaging to health and fattening. Although it relaxes your mind it acts as a stimulant (like tea and coffee) on your adrenal system, which is stressful for your body.

★ *Smoking.* May feel like a relaxant but is actually a stimulant. Expensive, smelly and damaging to health.

★ *Caffeine.* The stimulant contained in the three most popular drinks (apart from alcohol) worldwide: Coca-Cola, coffee and tea. It won't relax you but it's not quite as disastrous healthwise as smoking and alcohol.

★ *Overeating and undereating.* Has no long-term effect on stress other than to add to it by causing weight gain or illness.

* ★ *Overwork.* Has a short-term distracting effect but increases stress in the long run.
* ★ *Other drugs.* Expensive and may be damaging to health and relationships.

None of the above will actually cure stress. All of them will take your mind off it briefly. In the long term, quick fixes increase the pressure and some of them will make you ill.

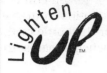 *The alternative to these quick fixes is a simple process called relaxation. It's easy to do, but takes a little preparation before you're ready to start.*

PUTTING MORE EFFORT INTO RELAXATION

Relaxation is the only sure-fire, long-term method of coping with stress. It's cheap, it's not antisocial and it doesn't damage your health. And it's the perfect substitute for eating when you aren't hungry.

It sounds obvious. So why are dysfunctional eating and chemical fixes still such popular stress busters? Probably because relaxation takes a little bit more effort. Most quick-fix techniques – especially ones like overeating, which we've been practising since we were children – work instantly for everybody.

LASTING CHANGE TAKES LONGER

 Last week we started with some basic breathing techniques. They're very simple but they take time. In fact, all relaxation techniques take time, energy and effort to get started. And before you can make some of them work for you, you have to get to know yourself better.

If you're thinking 'Oh, no, here comes the difficult bit, I knew there was going to be something about Lighten Up I wouldn't want to do . . .' don't panic; give it a chance. Learning to relax and get comfortable with yourself isn't difficult – but it isn't instant either. Lasting changes take longer but it's worth it. Here's the first stage:

 Take a moment to ask yourself:

★ What situations do you find stressful in terms of the hassles, irritations and glitches that get to you on a daily basis? We aren't talking about big stuff like death, marriage and moving house. Just the usual annoyances and exasperations of a typical day (or week).

....

★ Choose five of these and write them down in your Diary.

....

★ How do these situations make you feel? Do you get hot, cold, anxious, cross, aroused, angry, depressed?

....

★ How do you respond to feeling this way? Do you overeat, drink, smoke, take drugs, take it out on someone, store it up inside, undereat or overwork? See if you can come up with more than two techniques that you habitually use. If you've included any of the quick fixes (like alcohol), be prepared to start eliminating them over the next few weeks or months.

....

★ How might you respond differently under conditions that normally wind you up?

....

....

Next week I'll be introducing some relaxation techniques, but in the meantime carry on using the most important relaxation technique you'll ever learn: exercise. It's a simple matter of reversing the normal process and relaxing your mind while you exercise your body. You've been doing it for the past five weeks already and, as your body becomes fitter and stronger, your mind will learn to let go and relax.

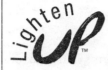 *Using exercise as a relaxation technique is like comfort-eating in reverse. It burns fat and makes you feel better.*

LISTEN TO YOUR BODY

The secret of relaxation is the same as the secret of being slim. It's about listening for the cues your body gives you and responding by giving your body what it needs. Get into the habit of listening and you will know when you're hungry and when you aren't. And you'll also know when you need exercise, when you need rest, and when you need to relax and do some deep breathing.

By this stage many of you have all the tools you need to live a healthy life. Some of them are already second nature and you instinctively pick them up whenever you find you need them. You're ready to shift your focus away from understanding the tools and healthy eating plans, and to start trusting the feedback you get from yourself.

Your body knows genetically, from birth, how to keep you at the perfect weight. It may not be *your* idea of the perfect weight because icons of beauty are rarely average in height, weight or appearance, meaning that most of the population can *never* naturally look like the people they most admire. The perfect weight for you may not be catwalk thin, but it won't be Mr Blobby either.

As a baby you refused to eat when you weren't hungry but, over the years, you learned to override this instinct. Your body never stopped sending you the messages about how much, when and what to eat, but you stopped listening.

If you're a leopard, you can't suddenly decide to make a fashion statement by joining up your spots and making them into stripes. You can't fight your genetic design. But although they *know* that, many people don't want to accept it. Normal eating and dieting are incompatible. Normal eaters eat regular meals. They don't worry about food and their diet tends to be very varied. They don't worry about their body weight either.

Life is for living and every day is full of potential that needs to be realised. Those new daily habits you've been playing around with will give you the feedback that'll help you stay happy and balanced.

So, loosen up a little, be flexible, listen to what your body is telling you and act accordingly.

Intuition

In Chapter Four we mentioned a study at Pennsylvania State University in 1999, which found that normal-weight men with no hang-ups about their weight have an inbuilt, subconscious calorie counter.[1] Well, most babies and young children have this too. It's also called your intuition – or messages from your subconscious mind.

People who are overweight have become very good at ignoring their internal signals and tend to respond to external signals instead. The aim of exercises like the Hunger Scale and Think Before You Eat is to get you to reverse this process. Of course, it won't happen overnight. If you've been driven by messages from the outside world for a long time, it will take effort to shut them out. And you'll need to start listening hard if you are going to pick up on those long-ignored internal cues.

 How many of these do you do regularly?

★ Checking the Hunger Scale before you eat.
★ Thinking Before You Eat. Are you really thinking internally

1 Barbara Rolls, Penn State University, 1999.

---

about what's going on inside you and what would feel good inside you?

★ Using the Fat Jar. If you're tempted to eat but aren't sure if it's really what you want, take a Fat Burning Pill instead. Put on your walking shoes and go for a fifteen-minute brisk walk. Getting your body moving is like an all-systems alert – after a little comfortable exercise you'll find your mind is much more in tune with how you really feel. Also, exercise doesn't immediately make you feel hungry – in fact, it tends to be a short-term appetite suppressant.

★ Using your Lighten Up Diary. If you don't know what you want, try writing the question down – on today's Diary page. It's almost impossible not to get some kind of an answer to the question forming in your mind once you've actually written it down.

If there's anything on this list that you aren't doing every day, put it in your Diary as a 'must do reminder' every day for the next week.

We are taught to override the common sense we were born with at an early age. Children are discouraged from running around because it's safer indoors, they're given sweets for comfort instead of real food for growth, they're told to accept the rules rather than thinking for themselves – so it's not surprising they turn into adults with unhealthy lifestyles.

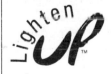 *Take yourself seriously. Everything your body is telling you could be useful.*

THE LIGHTEN UP DIARY

New Notes

★ Look out for your own pressure points this week. Notice where and when you are vulnerable. Don't comment or criticise, just write them down.

★ Which of the healthy cooking suggestions on pages 246–7 are you going to adopt this week? Write them down.
★ Do you have a potentially dangerous social situation this week? Write down which SAS technique you're going to use.
★ What happens when you feel stressed and you think you might resort to a quick fix like alcohol or food? Do you go for your usual solution, or do you substitute something else: a displacement activity, some deep breathing, a Fat-burning Pill or even a Feel Good Fitness session perhaps?

Carry On

★ using your Food Profile to get some feedback about whether you are eating a balanced diet;
★ noticing what you do when you have a little lapse and don't take any Fat-burning Pills for a few days or drink too much beer;
★ putting a congratulatory note in the Diary every time you eat slowly without doing something else at the same time;
★ using the Hunger Scale, and note down where you are on the scale in the middle of a meal as well as before it.

CHALLENGES

★ Aim to do at least three Feel Good Fitness sessions and add a fourth if you didn't already do that last week.
★ Try out some of the healthy cooking suggestions and use some of the recipes at the back of the book.
★ Spend this week being your own best friend, giving yourself encouraging messages, listening to your body and treating yourself with respect.
★ Experiment with a new way of increasing your activity levels – a new Feel Good Fitness activity perhaps, something you haven't done before like dancing or rollerblading.
★ If you are still getting rid of old, unwanted eating patterns, be sure to give yourself credit for all your victories, large or small.
★ Run either the Movie exercise or the Open Door exercise in your mind a couple of times this week.

CHECKLIST FOR WEEK SIX

Weekly checklist

You're down to your last eating pattern! Which is it?

....

On which four days are you going to do your Feel Good Fitness sessions? Write them here:

Feel Good Fitness session 1: ....

Feel Good Fitness session 2: ....

Feel Good Fitness session 3: ....

Feel Good Fitness session 4: ....

Daily checklist	Day 1	Day 2	Day 3	Day 4	Day 5	Day 6	Day 7
Do the Hunger Scale at least three times a day	☐	☐	☐	☐	☐	☐	☐
Think Before You Eat	☐	☐	☐	☐	☐	☐	☐
First Fat Burning Pill	☐	☐	☐	☐	☐	☐	☐
Second Fat Burning Pill	☐	☐	☐	☐	☐	☐	☐
First Affirmation session	☐	☐	☐	☐	☐	☐	☐
Second Affirmation session	☐	☐	☐	☐	☐	☐	☐
Breathing exercises	☐	☐	☐	☐	☐	☐	☐
Do a 2-minute Worry Dump	☐	☐	☐	☐	☐	☐	☐
Go to sleep on a positive thought	☐	☐	☐	☐	☐	☐	☐
The Lighten Up Diary	☐	☐	☐	☐	☐	☐	☐

My goal for the rest of the programme is:

....

WEEK SEVEN
OF THE
EIGHT-WEEK
COURSE

HOW ARE YOU DOING?

We asked you to be aware of a lot of things last week. Some of them will be ideas, or techniques, that you're taking for granted and doing automatically. There will be a few that you're not too sure about and maybe aren't right for you quite yet. And there will be some that you're still working on.

LAST WEEK'S LIGHTEN UP DIARY
AND CHALLENGES

★ How is your Food Profile looking at the moment?
★ How much sugar, hidden fat and convenience food are you eating?
★ Have you added in some more fresh fruit and vegetables?
★ Are you getting your vitamins and minerals and essential fatty acids from any new sources – like nuts and seeds, for example?

★ Are you drinking plenty of water?

★ Did you experiment with some more healthy ways of cooking food and try out some new recipes?

★ Where are you on the Hunger Scale when you eat?

★ Did you enjoy your four Feel Good Fitness sessions this week? Are you doing the same kind of exercise as when you started or are you trying some new ideas. Whether it's ballroom dancing or martial arts, it doesn't matter as long as you do it and enjoy it. How about the Fat Jar and the Fat Burning Pills? There's a daily dose of two on your Checklist but a lot of people find at this stage that they're doing more. Once you get the idea of a more active lifestyle you might find yourself doing things you would never have dreamed of doing before (like going to work in trainers and keeping your shoes in your desk).

★ Are you still using Think Before You Eat and sometimes writing down the food you reject as well as the food you select? Has this shown you anything about how you might have changed?

★ How did you feel about being your own best friend for a week? Have you been giving yourself credit for everything you get right? How do you feel about learning to listen to what your body wants you to do and eat, and trusting your intuition?

★ Did you have any opportunities to see how you cope with resisting social pressures to eat?

★ Are you still eating when you're stressed, or bored or lonely? Did any of the displacement activities or breathing and relaxation techniques help you to resist the temptation?

★ Have you experimented with using exercise instead of eating as an instant relaxation technique?

★ Did any other old eating patterns bite the dust? Often, when people have been keeping the Diary for a few weeks, they are surprised at just how many eating (and other) patterns have come to light that they never noticed before.

★ What did you choose to do this week – was it the Movie or the Open Door visualisation? If it was the Movie, did you use your Affirmation as part of the exercise? And are you still saying your Affirmations to yourself at least twice a day?

Are You Ready?

As you read through this chapter, remember you are getting ready to take what works with you into the future. There won't be a new chapter every week for the rest of your life telling you what to do. From now on you're instinctively going to know what to do and this week you can start thinking about the techniques and ideas you'll keep and the ones you'll dip into from time to time.

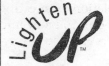 **WEEK SEVEN**

★ We start this week by encouraging you to look at your energy levels. Energy is one of the most important progress indicators when you're losing weight and changing to a healthier lifestyle.

★ We've talked about food groups over the past few weeks and this week we're going to be looking at the process that deals with that food – your digestion.

★ The Changing Your Association with Food and the Sound Effects exercises are designed to help you get rid of – or control your reaction to – any unhealthy foods that are still throwing your Food Profile out of balance.

★ Food shopping that doesn't sabotage your slimming

★ More relaxation techniques to help you respond to stress without overeating or drinking.

★ Update your beliefs, paying attention to what you want and how you're achieving it, taking responsibility for the action that's going to help you achieve your goal.

★ Respect: upgrading your self-image.

ENERGY LEVELS

Your energy levels are a great guide to your health and state of mind. Filling in the chart on pages 266–7 for a week may give you some very interesting insights into why you feel tired or energetic, why you seem to achieve more on some days than on others and why you feel hungry when you do. Tracking your energy levels can tell you a lot about whether you're eating the right food and taking the right exercise.

 Copy one of the blank graphs into your Diary for every day of next week. Keep track of your energy levels and see if there's any correlation with eating and exercise (or anything else you do). You may find that certain foods make you sleepy while others give you energy. You may discover lots of other patterns too.

We often aren't aware that there are definable, predictable patterns in our energy levels and that we can control them more effectively than we think: what we eat, whether or not we exercise and, of course, whether or not we're ill will all make a difference. Being more aware of all these factors will help you work with your body, rather than against it. Every day, draw your energy line on the graph and, whenever you get a dip or a rise, make a note of what you were doing just before. Did you eat? Did you go for a walk? Did you get upset about something? Stress is often mistaken for high energy – but that's the adrenaline effect. When it wears off, a very lethargic low is likely to follow.

Just keep track and discover what gives you energy and what drains it away. We want you to be more aware of how you feel and why, so that you can take more control over your own life. This is an experiment, so be patient and remember, once you know what's happening, you have the power to change it. When you know how different foods and activity patterns affect you, it will be much easier to start making the changes that will help you stay alert and energetic during the day and fall easily asleep at night.

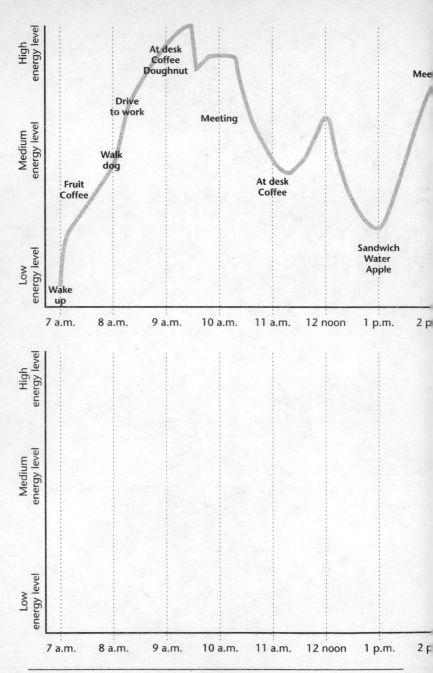

LIGHTEN UP

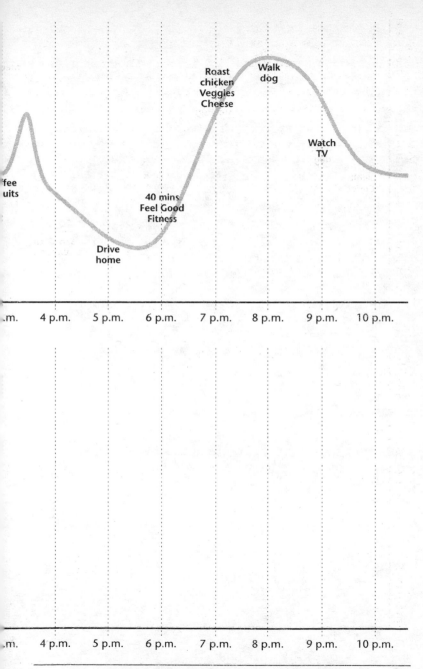

fee
uits

Coffee
Biscuits

Drive
home

40 mins
Feel Good
Fitness

Roast
chicken
Veggies
Cheese

Walk
dog

Watch
TV

.m. 4 p.m. 5 p.m. 6 p.m. 7 p.m. 8 p.m. 9 p.m. 10 p.m.

.m. 4 p.m. 5 p.m. 6 p.m. 7 p.m. 8 p.m. 9 p.m. 10 p.m.

DIGESTION

If you'd like more information about food groups, you'll find everything you need in Chapter Seventeen. This week, instead of talking about food, we want to draw your attention to what your body does with it.

A lot of people take their digestive system for granted until it causes them pain or stops working properly – and that happens quite a lot, especially as we get older. Digestive problems are very common, which is hardly surprising, given how complex the digestive process is.

Although digestion is automatic, there's a lot we can do to make it more comfortable and efficient. It's easy to put food in your mouth, chew it and then forget about it – but as far as your body's concerned the hardest part is still to come. After you've swallowed it, food passes into your stomach, where it starts being broken down into nutrients that your body can absorb, and then into the small intestine. The remaining waste matter is stored in the colon ready for elimination. That's a lot of plumbing and a lot of complicated chemistry, but most people take more care of their cars or their homes than they do of their digestive tracts.

WHAT YOU EAT

When someone says they're finding something hard to digest, they could be referring to food or to ideas. The Lighten Up programme is full of positive ideas that will make it easier for you to change your life. And you can apply the same principle to your stomach. If you eat good natural food that isn't overcooked, or processed, or full of additives, and is easy to digest, you're less likely to have problems.

FIBRE

Whole diets have been built around fibre – and by all accounts some of them were pretty antisocial. The idea behind these diets is presumably to keep food moving through your system so fast that you won't absorb it. That's not a healthy way to live. Your digestive system is designed to ensure you *do* absorb all the nutrients your body needs to keep you fit and healthy – and you will only ever be permanently slim if you are fit and healthy as well. Unfortunately, many slimming programmes blatantly disregard this principle and encourage people to eat an unbalanced diet that actually stresses the digestive system.

Eating a lot of fibre won't in itself make you slim but it's useful to understand how it works to aid your digestive process. There are two types of fibre: soluble and insoluble.

★ *Insoluble fibre* (in many fruit and vegetables) passes through your gut unchanged, carrying some fat with it and speeding up the digestive process.
★ *Soluble fibre* (in beans, oats, barley, broccoli, prunes, apples and citrus fruits) helps lower both cholesterol and blood sugar levels.

Eating plenty of fibre helps you stay healthy and keeps your digestive processes running smoothly.

HOW YOU EAT

Your digestion has two functions:

★ to break food into bits small enough to be absorbed from the gut into the bloodstream;
★ to convert food into a form that can be used by your body cells.

Your body has more chance of doing this efficiently if you

★ take your time, eat slowly and chew your food properly;
★ give your system a break, don't eat constantly and don't overeat.

Being kind to your digestion has a slimming side-effect. It will slow down your eating so that you can

★ register the 'I'm full' signals before you finish a meal;
★ get a better idea of how particular foods are making you feel.

DO THIS **next time you eat:** Think about the amazing process happening inside you, the way your body's going to use the food you just ate to keep you slim, fit and healthy. Be respectful of this process and be aware of how the food you eat is making you feel.

LOSING YOUR TASTE
FOR YOUR FAVOURITE FOOD

You're starting to think about the broader, long-term picture of you, the exercise you take, the food you eat and how it keeps you slim, fit and healthy. Is there anything that still seems obviously out of balance? When you look at your Food Profile, is the Foods to Focus On circle looking bigger and fuller than the circle at the bottom? Towards the end of the course, we often find that people who are doing really well with their healthy eating plan still have one or two foods in the Foods to Limit circle at the bottom that they just can't give up.

Of course, for some people it's easy. They might have a Magnum now and again, or the odd glass of wine, but it's an occasional pleasure not a habit. If that's true for you, then you might want to skip the next couple of exercises. But if you have a food addiction you still can't shake, it's time to take drastic action.

So what, if anything, is still throwing your Food Profile out of balance? Is there something you find really hard to resist? Chocolate, crisps, or Coca-Cola perhaps? If you think you have a dependency relationship with a particular food, you can change your association with it – forever if you want to. Of course, the Think Before You Eat exercise is helping you by now to choose the foods your body needs and likes, and you may already have been able to eliminate most of the junk from your diet. But if you need a bit of extra help with something that still has a real hold on you, the next two exercises will help you break the spell.

Before we start, stop and think. Are there any particularly sugary or fattening foods you would like to cut out of your diet? Write them down.

....

....

Sound Effects

DO THIS NOW Point with one finger to a part of your body you would like to be slimmer.

Think of the food or foods you're still eating but would like to give up, something fattening and sugary perhaps, or heavy and fried. And again, point to the part of your body where you think those foods will go when you eat them.

For the next three weeks, every time you look at food, pause for a moment and think about whether it's the sort of food your body will digest comfortably to give you energy and make you feel good. Is it the sort of food that would make your body say 'Mm' and 'Ah' with appreciation?

Or is it something you don't think your body needs: heavy, fatty, over-processed, sweetened food perhaps? Is it the sort of food that would make your body go 'Yuck.'

You don't have to say this out loud – though you can if you want to. Just be careful not to embarrass yourself: one lady once forgot where she was and shouted 'Yuck' at the dessert trolley in a restaurant. So it's possibly something that's best practised in the privacy of your own home.

Save Sound Effects for the real food baddies and remember that some of the foods we think we want won't do anything for our health and well-being. Foods that are refined and full of chemicals, sugar and fat are difficult to digest and can make you feel bloated and tired. So missing out on them isn't really a big loss, is it?

All you're doing is building some new and helpful associations, which will make slimming easier. After all, the associations you have with food are just things you've learned: babies aren't instinctively drawn to Mars bars. These ideas will help you make some useful changes and you can use the Sound Effects to help you with the next exercise: Changing Your Association with Food.

Changing Your Association With Food

This is a very simple exercise, but it takes a bit of practice. If it doesn't work first time, come back to it. The aim is to get you to associate a really disgusting taste and smell with something you would normally be crazy about – like Crème Eggs, for example, or bacon sandwiches. Whatever it is that you normally just can't resist, let's see if we can ruin it for you and put you off it for life.

This technique is very effective, so before you start, ask yourself if you really want to give up the toffee crunch (or whatever it is for you).

 Find a quiet, comfortable place where you won't be disturbed and get someone to read the exercise out for you. If you don't have anyone handy, do what you did with the Open Door in Week One. Read it once, just to get a feel for it, then read it out again as if you were helping somebody else with it. Pretend you're demonstrating it in front of an imaginary group. Do that twice. Then settle down, read yourself the instructions and do what you tell yourself to do. It's not a good one to try on the tube home from work, or in the pub on a Saturday night because the expression on your face at the end is going to give you away.

1 First close your eyes and take a couple of deep breaths.
2 Think of the food that you would like to stop eating.
3 Picture this food in front of you. If you can taste it and smell it as soon as you picture it, that's usually a sign that you have a strong association with it.
4 Make the image of the food into a framed picture.
5 Push the picture a few feet further away from you. Use your arms and do the actions.
6 If the picture is in colour, turn down the brightness so that it's dark, or black and white.

7 Hold this dull picture in your mind. Think of a smell you really hate and breathe it deep into your lungs. If it's not bad enough, find a worse one.

8 With that smell in your nose, think of a taste you find really revolting. Maybe something you hated as a child.

9 Roll the taste round your mouth (if you can bear it). You don't have to swallow.

10 Keeping the foul taste in your mouth, bring back the dull picture.

11 With the picture in front of you, surround it with the obnoxious smell you conjured up.

12 Add the 'Yuck' noise you were using in the last exercise.

13 Take the food out of the picture and bring it towards you, smelling the obnoxious smell and tasting the revolting taste you added to it.

14 Go on, treat yourself. Have a bite. Or would you rather not?

There are all sorts of variations on this, including a man who imagined his chips covered in dog food and a girl who made cheesecake taste like tripe.

I'm sure you've got the idea by now, so feel free to be as disgusting as you like. If you want to recondition yourself for total success and permanent pleasure, put yourself through this little bit of pain each day at first. Do this exercise daily for the rest of this week and then use it whenever you feel a particular kind of food is getting a hold on you. The more you practise this exercise, the more powerful it will become.

Do you like it enough to wear it?

Making Mars bars smell like furniture polish and learning to say 'Yuck' when you see a chocolate mousse are very effective techniques. At Lighten Up we hear from people who practised those responses years ago and still find them useful. A more straightforward approach, of course, is just to argue back.

When a packet of crisps begs you to eat it, tell it to shut up.

But, if you want to make it a bit stronger than that, feel free. Whatever it takes to make that temptation go away. You don't have to be polite to a Banoffi pie.

Another approach when you can hear the ice-cream calling is to ask yourself: 'Do I like it enough to wear it?'

It's not a new idea, but it's such a powerful one that I've even used it on television. It was the *Lorraine Kelly Show* a couple of years ago and she happened to have a chocolate cake handy, so I spread it liberally over my thighs in front of the camera. It wasn't an appealing sight but a lot of people who watched that morning tell me that whenever they look at chocolate cake now they ask themselves whether they really want to wear it.

If you want to stay slim you can give yourself a lot of help. Reshuffle your positive and negative associations so that exercise and healthy eating seem easy and fun, and slobbing and stuffing seem painful and uncomfortable.

If you're forcing yourself into a lifestyle you hate you'll never keep it up. Use pleasure as your ally. Laugh at yourself when you get it wrong and try to hold some compellingly attractive images of yourself in your mind the rest of the time.

 Think of your favourite fattening food. The one you want to eat less of. Imagine it spread over the bit of your body you'd rather have less of. Make the picture as clear and bright as you can and file it away so that you can pull it out next time that particular food starts ordering you around.

THINK BEFORE YOU SHOP

A more practical approach to staying slim is to go food shopping – not as a displacement activity, or even a form of exercise (although it can be both of those).

IT'S TOUGH GOING SHOPPING

What's so hard about shopping? Well, a trip to a superstore can be the fastest way to sabotage a weight loss initiative. You need strength and determination to survive and, like most military operations, it needs precise planning if you are to succeed.

Preparing for a shopping trip takes skill and patience. Supermarkets, not surprisingly, are designed with the profit of the shareholders rather than the health of the shoppers in mind. The good thing about them is that there is plenty of choice and the organic sections are getting larger all the time. The Think Before You Eat strategy applies to shopping as well and Thinking Before You Shop is something you can quickly train yourself to do. You can eventually train other members of your household to do it as well, but don't be too ambitious; start on yourself.

Big food stores are often arranged and then rearranged just to confuse you. As soon as you've memorised one layout it gets changed so you end up looking at things you never planned to buy. However, the fruit and veggies are usually at the front as your resistance to buying is higher at the start of the shopping trip and fresh produce is often a lower profit margin item because of its short shelf life.

The bright, sugary fattening foods and the alcohol are normally in the last aisles you come to, when you're tired and you'll buy anything just so you can go home. But there's nothing to stop you starting at the far end and working back to the fruit and veg, is there? What's more, if you balance the bananas and tomatoes on top of the rice and cans of beans, instead of letting them get squashed at the bottom of your trolley, they'll look much more appetising when you get them home.

HOW TO TELL WHEN YOU'RE READY TO GO SHOPPING

★ You have planned your meals for the next week.
★ You have made a list.
★ You have your magnifying glass to read the labels so you can reject the ones with too many chemicals.
★ You're looking forward to buying some fresh foods and you don't mind putting in a bit of extra time on the preparation (check out some of the recipes at the back of the book).
★ You have just had a meal.

 Plan your next food-shopping trip. Decide what you'll need for a whole week and take a look at the recipes and store cupboard suggestions at the back of the book.

RELAXATION

Why do we spend so much time on the Lighten Up programme talking about breathing and relaxation techniques instead of calories? The reason for this is simple.

PEOPLE OFTEN OVEREAT BECAUSE THEY CAN'T RELAX

There are much better ways to cope with stress, boredom and the general aggravation of life than eating – or drinking. Especially if anxiety about your appearance is the problem that drives you to drink or eat: you'll end up fatter and more miserable than ever and you'll probably reach out for yet another glass of wine and plate of chips.

You already know that exercise is a great way of coping with stress and it makes you slimmer at the same time. The displacement activities we've talked about are also a brilliant idea. But the best substitute for eating when you aren't hungry is to *relax*. And the bonus is that it makes it much *much* easier for you to tell where you are on the Hunger Scale and to Think Before You Eat.

A lot of people take much better care of their cars than they do of themselves and I can't think of anyone who believes their car will run perfectly if they just put oil, petrol and water into it regularly. We know there are times when a car needs a complete service.

The rapid pace of modern life means we don't pay much attention to our occasional need to take a break and give ourselves an overhaul. Of course, we probably take a holiday once in a while. But holidays don't always mean rest and recreation for body and mind. They can just as easily mean a week or two of no-holds-barred eating and drinking, accompanied by extreme over-exercising or under-exercising. The result is returning to work feeling mentally and physically worse than before.

So far we've been talking about the minimum care you need to give your mind and body by eating sensibly, exercising regularly and being kind to yourself. But you can do better than that. What is all the stress in your life telling you? It's telling you you need to practise the art of relaxation and learn to let all the tension go.

Until now you've been learning the proper way to service your body and mind and now you're ready to acquire the wonderful habit of relaxation, which renews, regenerates and helps you cope with stress. Relaxation calms you down, gives you endless energy and allows you to free yourself from external pressures. It gives you time to daydream and renew your focus on becoming slimmer, fitter and healthier.

Take a deep breath

Remember the breathing exercises? There's no time like the present, so why not pause, right now, and take a deep breath, in through your nose. Count to four as you breathe in and count to four again as you slowly breathe out once more through your nose. How does that feel? Make each breath slightly deeper than the last.

Taking a deep breath is the easiest and one of the most effective ways to relax. It's one of the reasons a lot of people smoke – that's the only time they take a really deep breath. It's just a pity it's also highly toxic. Breathe deeply more often, especially when you are starting to feel stressed, angry or worried. Maybe the old saying 'take a deep breath and count to ten' has got some truth in it after all.

Adjust your surroundings

Find a calm place in your mind. You could be doing something like walking, taking a bath or having a massage while you do this. Picture a warm, sandy beach, a cosy fireside, a quiet forest clearing, or a moonlit veranda on a hot night. Allow harmony, peace and quiet voices. Choose a positive idea (like being slimmer) and keep it in your head. Imagine you can hear some of your favourite music playing and tell yourself a story about something you would like to happen.

Copy the cat

Tune in to another creature's ability to relax. Watch the fish, stroke the cat, go horse riding. Human beings behave like harmless parasites with certain animals. We absorb their calm and steady breathing, and their inability to worry.

But be careful. It can work in reverse. Nervous animals and

stressed, aggressive people transmit negative energy and raise your blood pressure if you get close to them.

Take a peaceful view

Think of something that made you feel good recently. Relive the experience and try to pinpoint that good feeling as much as you can. Now visualise yourself in the future, feeling that same feeling in lots of different situations. Some of these situations might be ones in which you wouldn't normally feel good. Let your imagination fill in the gaps. The technical name for this technique is daydreaming.

Go for a massage

Give yourself a regular treat. Get somebody else to relax you. Massage, reflexology and aromatherapy are all great relaxers because they work through more than one sense at a time. Touch and smell together can be powerful relaxants.

Physical activity

You already know this but we're putting it in again because it's so important. Exercise works for a lot of people because it uses up stress hormones in a natural way, restoring the body to a healthy balance. Dancing, gardening, jogging or walking the dog, to name but a few.

Find relaxers that work for you and indulge, often.

Chilling out

★ Find a quiet place where you can sit without being disturbed for ten minutes.

★ Sit comfortably, with your back straight, facing forward and both feet flat on the floor. Turn the lighting down or off.

★ Focus on your breathing as you notice the gentle rise and fall of your chest. Follow your breath in through your nose, right into your body and back out through your nose.

★ Follow your breath now with a little more concentration. Be aware of the air streaming in through your nostrils and filling your lungs. Imagine you can see the air being drawn down deeper into your body, filling it with life.

★ Keep your breathing at the front of your mind so that you become aware of it without thinking about it.

★ If any thoughts creep into your head, acknowledge them and let them go. You might wonder why certain things come into your mind, and feel obliged to go with a thought. Push it away. Imagine putting all those thoughts into the bin or down the waste disposal unit and bring your attention back to your breath.

★ Begin to count your breaths at the end of every outward breath. Hear yourself saying the number.

★ If you lose your place or forget the number it doesn't matter. Just start again at the beginning. The counting is simply to focus your attention on your breathing.

★ You might find that some days your mind is more active than others, but just expect whatever you experience and notice the deep relaxation and peace you feel.

HOW CHILLING OUT WORKS

Chilling out – and a hundred other very similar techniques – is best practised before you need it. Of course, you can still use it when the pressure hits. But it works much better if you do it regularly when you aren't stressed, when everything is fine(ish) and you can take that time to be alone with yourself. In fact, when you make a habit of chilling out, those feelings of unbearable tension probably won't be as common as they used to be.

By practising the chilling-out technique every day, you will learn to be more positive and get better and better at coping with stressful situations. You will also become more relaxed and your general health and well-being will improve.

Chilling out teaches your brain to do exactly the opposite of what it does when you become stressed. It teaches greater control of your thoughts and makes it easier to have deeper levels of rest. Imagine how good you'll feel when you stop worrying about things you can't change.

Practising this technique trains your mind to focus on just one thing at a time. Which is not something we naturally do. Your ability to relax at will increases as you teach yourself to manage your thoughts and dissolve stress and tension.

This exercise is often met with resistance and the resistance comes from inside us. Our minds are normally active and that's what they're used to. It's the mental status quo. The chilling-out technique teaches the mind to behave counter-intuitively, so it's bound to take a little while. Everybody wants instant results, which is why quick-fix remedies are so popular. Chilling out is not a quick-fix remedy. If you want it to work for you, you need to put it in the same place as your new commitment to a more active lifestyle. It's something you will do regularly, until it becomes second nature to you. And you'll do it because you want to feel permanently relaxed and calm. It's such a simple, straightforward way of relaxing that you might ask yourself how it could possibly be so effective. The answer is to practise it and see for yourself. All you need to do is give yourself 10 minutes morning and evening. If you like it, you can gradually increase this to 20 minutes over the next few weeks.

It is better to practise this routine before you eat, but it is totally compatible with exercise. In fact, some people get the same result through exercise alone. But you won't know if this technique will be a regular habit for you until you give it a fair trial. And even if it's not going to be part of your daily life, it's well worth learning the breathing technique for use in stressful situations. Whenever you find yourself under pressure, just take a moment to follow your breath and let yourself relax as you gradually regain control of your feelings.

WHAT MAKES YOU THINK YOU'RE GETTING THINNER?

Do you remember the bit about beliefs in Chapter One? If you've read all the chapters between then and now, you've been doing and thinking a lot of things that will strengthen your belief in your own success. You have been adding legs to your belief in your own slimness as you've tested the techniques, added more exercise to your daily routine and focused on your Food Profile.

DO THIS NOW So if you really believe you can be slimmer now, what is supporting this belief?

I'm doing at least three Feel Good Fitness sessions every week.
I'm being patient.
I'm being positive.
I'm thinking before I eat.
I'm using my Affirmations.
I'm checking the Hunger Scale.
I'm thinking before I buy.
I'm eating a balanced diet.
I'm filling in the Food Profile.
I've slowed down my eating.
I'm setting myself outcomes.
I'm focusing on my goal.
I'm drinking plenty of water.
I'm writing down what I eat.
I'm taking my Fat Burning Pills.
I'm eating more nutritious foods.
I can refuse food if I'm not really hungry.
I'm learning from everything that has happened to me.
I'm relaxing instead of eating when I get upset.

What else are you doing to support your belief in yourself as a slim person?

....

....

....

....

....

....

....

....

Attention

Whatever you pay attention to, and what you decide to think about, affects how you feel and what you do. We all move towards whatever we regularly, consistently focus on and imagine. Occasional thoughts may flit through our minds. But it's only the regular, persistent offenders that can ruin our lives.

 Ask yourself:

'What have I been thinking about most, today and every day for the past week?'

....

'Have these thoughts been helpful and encouraging and optimistic? Or not?'

....

Most people think about what others think or what others are doing. True champions tend to be much more concerned with themselves and what they can control. Every thought can have two consequences it either moves you closer to your dream of being slimmer or takes you further away.

The first step towards positive change is to start thinking it's possible. Most of us don't seem to think that way and maybe that's why only 10 per cent of people who buy a book like this read past the first chapter and fewer than 10 per cent of people bother to write down their goals.

The second step towards positive change is to put positive thoughts into action. Why do so few people live the life of their dreams and look the way they want to look? Because it takes effort and action. If you don't follow up your dreams by taking action, you still won't get what you want.

Let's look at another 10 per cent to illustrate this one. Everybody knows that, in order to be slimmer, fitter and healthier, we need to be physically active. Thousands of people in the UK would like to be slimmer, fitter and healthier than they are – so why is it that only 10 per cent of the population actually make the effort to take enough exercise?

Very few people actually walk their talk. Yet that is all they need to do.

Walk your talk

 This is a quick review of your progress to date:

1 Who do you think is responsible for you becoming slimmer?

....

2 Are you clear about exactly what you want? Can you picture it, hear it and feel it in your mind? Or is it still a little out of focus?

....

3 How much do you really want to be slimmer? What will you get out of being slimmer? Exactly how will your life be different?

....

4 How will you feel about yourself when it happens?

....

5 How strong is your belief that you can be slimmer? What evidence do you have for it? (This might include exercise, changes in eating habits, more self-respect . . .)

....

6 Are you ready and willing to continue taking action?

....

If your belief in your ability to make your changes is still a little shaky, how many of these could you brush up on?

★ Exercising regularly so that it becomes an enjoyable part of your daily life.

* ★ Learning from your mistakes instead of blaming yourself for them.
* ★ Drinking more water and less tea, coffee and soft drinks.
* ★ Filling in more of the top Food Profile circle than the bottom.
* ★ Eating only when your body tells you that you really are hungry.
* ★ Running the Hunger Scale and Think Before You Eat more regularly.
* ★ Being much nicer to yourself.

WILLING AND RESPONSIBLE

Of course, these aren't questions you can answer quickly. Take the time to think them through. You are looking to find out whether you are really ready to change and become slimmer, fitter and healthier than you have been before. It all depends on the strength of your belief in your ability to change and whether the change is right for you.

Some beliefs have stronger foundations than others. Once you've built the belief, you can set about reinforcing the foundations. You are probably getting slimmer and you believe that you will be a slim person in the future.

A lot of people go through life blaming others when things go wrong. We all do it sometimes. When you give responsibility for your life to others you are depriving yourself of a precious opportunity to learn. Because you can't learn from other people's mistakes as easily as you can from your own.

If you really want something, first you have to be willing to perform all the actions required to take you there. Second, you've got to understand that you alone are responsible for doing whatever it takes to get where you want to go. This is a very liberating attitude: it frees you up from blaming others and allows you to focus on yourself and do what you need to do to achieve your goal.

Rephrasing it

We've talked before about the language you use and the way you talk to yourself. Have you been making some changes in the way you talk to yourself now? Even in the eighth week of a Lighten Up course we sometimes catch people telling us they're 'trying really hard'. The habits of a lifetime are difficult to break, but this is the language of failure and you've got to stop using it.

People who truly want something don't use words like *must, should, ought, try,* or *persevere.* The minute you start talking to yourself in language like that you sow the seeds of doubt in your mind. Then the whole enterprise starts looking like really hard work. This is just a reminder – if you've got out of the habit of listening to what you say to yourself, get back into it for a while. And, if you catch yourself saying 'I ought', 'I hope', 'I should', and 'I might', tell yourself to 'shut up'.

RESPECT YOURSELF

This is a really key part of the Lighten Up programme. If you don't feel good about yourself, why on earth would you bother about making positive changes in your life?

THE IMAGE OF MADNESS

Nobody's born thinking they are ugly or believing their bum or their nose is too big. If you feel bad about your appearance it will be something you've learned over the years. Maybe other people put you down or maybe you did it for yourself, but somewhere along the line you started thinking you were sub-standard. Sadly, wherever these messages are coming from they are convincing an awful lot of people that they are physically sub-standard human beings.[1]

Now is the time to convince yourself that you're fine. Just because you don't look like Cindy Crawford doesn't mean you're not beautiful. You are as amazing as everybody else. Your heart has been beating for you since the day you were born. Your liver performs over 400 different jobs for you every day. Your digestive system sorts out all the junk you put inside yourself. Your body and mind are the most sophisticated pieces of equipment you will ever own. And you're unique.

1 A survey by *Top Santé* magazine in summer 2000 showed that only 1 per cent of women are happy with their whole body.

How do you behave when you're with someone you truly admire – a parent, teacher, mentor, priest, guru, leader, boss, colleague or friend? Don't you give them time, affection and even respect? You might disagree with them sometimes, but would you be constantly pointing out their every little defect? It's not very likely, is it?

★ Is your body worth respecting?

....

★ If not, why not?

....

★ If yes, why?

....

★ Would you like to respect your body more than you do?

....

TIPS FOR TREATING YOUR BODY WITH RESPECT

Put a tick against the things you've started to do more of over the past few weeks. Put a cross against the ones you *haven't* started yet . . . and then make sure you start doing them this week.

★ If your body tells you you're thirsty, drink.
If it tells you you're hungry, eat. ☐

★ Look after your body, spare-part surgery has a
long way to go. ☐

★ Say something nice to yourself when you wake up
in the morning and when you sign off at night. ☐

★ Eat healthy, fresh food. ☐

★ Keep moving. That's what you were designed for.
You know what happens to a bicycle chain when
you don't look after your bike and use it regularly. ☐

★ Cut down on the things you don't enjoy, increase
the things you do and make the things you've *got* to
do more fun. ☐

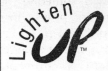

When you pause to do a mini-review like this, it's a good idea to get out your Diary and make some notes. Writing down the answers to questions, for example, often clarifies them.

THE LIGHTEN UP DIARY

New Notes

★ Copy the Energy Graph into your Diary for each day of the week and draw in your energy line. Then add in your exercise, your eating and whether you've used one of the relaxation techniques.

★ List your daily outcomes again as you did in Week Four and notice how they are helping you towards your goal.

★ Plan your meals for the week, write a list of the fresh foods you will need and also a basic store-cupboard list. We've dropped a couple of hints about writing purposeful shopping lists in Weeks Four and Five, so you may already have made a start. But if you haven't, now's the time. You may like to take a look at Chapter Nineteen first for some recipe ideas and a list of basic store-cupboard items.

★ Write down the belief you have about yourself being slimmer and list the actions you are taking which support that belief. Take into account your self-image at the moment – how do you really think you look right now? How much respect are you able to feel for yourself and the actions you are taking to become slimmer?

Carry On

★ filling in the Food Profile;

★ noting where you are on the Hunger Scale when you eat;

★ noting when you eat for reasons other than hunger (are there still some persistent patterns of eating you'd like to change?);

★ writing down the feelings you associate with food.

CHALLENGES

★ Shop for the week, having first made your list of fresh and store-cupboard foods.

★ We've added a couple of chilling-out sessions to your Checklist this week, but try some of the other relaxation techniques too. A different one every day would be a good idea.

★ Try yet another new form of exercise. There are plenty you can do by yourself, like cycling, running up and down stairs, swimming or working out to videos. And the classes and clubs you can join are almost unlimited: aerobics, t'ai chi, line dancing, gymnastics or perhaps a martial art to help keep the family in order. If you haven't already added in the extra one, make it your target to do at least four Feel Good Fitness sessions this week.

★ Be your own best friend for another week. At least. If you find yourself getting attached it could turn into the partnership of a lifetime.

CHECKLIST FOR WEEK SEVEN

Weekly checklist

On which four days are you going to do your Feel Good Fitness sessions? Write them here:

Feel Good Fitness session 1: ....

Feel Good Fitness session 2: ....

Feel Good Fitness session 3: ....

Feel Good Fitness session 4: ....

Daily checklist	Day 1	Day 2	Day 3	Day 4	Day 5	Day 6	Day 7
Sound Effects exercise	☐	☐	☐	☐	☐	☐	☐
Changing Your Association With Food	☐	☐	☐	☐	☐	☐	☐
First Chilling-out session	☐	☐	☐	☐	☐	☐	☐
Second Chilling-out session	☐	☐	☐	☐	☐	☐	☐
First Fat Burning Pill	☐	☐	☐	☐	☐	☐	☐
Second Fat Burning Pill	☐	☐	☐	☐	☐	☐	☐
First Affirmation session	☐	☐	☐	☐	☐	☐	☐
Second Affirmation session	☐	☐	☐	☐	☐	☐	☐
Visualisation – the Movie or the Open Door	☐	☐	☐	☐	☐	☐	☐
Think Before You Eat	☐	☐	☐	☐	☐	☐	☐
Think Before You Eat	☐	☐	☐	☐	☐	☐	☐
Think Before You Eat	☐	☐	☐	☐	☐	☐	☐

continued

Daily checklist (continued)	Day 1	Day 2	Day 3	Day 4	Day 5	Day 6	Day 7
Congratulating yourself on an achievement	☐	☐	☐	☐	☐	☐	☐
Energy Graph	☐	☐	☐	☐	☐	☐	☐
The Lighten Up Diary	☐	☐	☐	☐	☐	☐	☐

My goal for the rest of the programme is:

....

....

CHAPTER SIXTEEN

WEEK EIGHT
OF THE
EIGHT-WEEK
COURSE

HOW ARE YOU DOING?

Congratulations on getting this far! We hope you've had as much fun as we do in the eight-week evening classes. By now you're probably looking great and feeling fantastic – and well on your way to a slimmer, fitter and healthier you. In this, the final week of the course, we'll be giving you all the techniques for staying motivated that you're ever likely to need and showing you how to make Lighten Up a permanent part of your life.

Are You Ready?

As you go through this chapter, answer the questions quickly and honestly. There's no point in giving the answers you think you should give. The key to change is knowing where you're starting from. It doesn't matter *where* that is – but it is important to know.

When you come across one of those new, crucial pieces of brain software that we've already introduced you to – like the Hunger Scale or Think Before You Eat – remember to ask yourself whether you're doing it automatically yet.

Many of the basic principles of Lighten Up, like positive thinking and strong self-belief, are strategies that slim, successful people use without even thinking about it. They aren't magic and they aren't anything to do with thin genes or willpower. They are just simple techniques that you can learn if you want to.

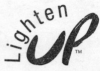 **FOR LIFE**

As this is the final week of the Lighten Up programme, you might reasonably be expecting a list of ultimate answers. In fact, what you're going to get is a list of the ultimate questions. You already know the answers – you've been discovering them for yourself during the past seven weeks of the programme. Just be sure that you have confidence in what you've learned so far and keep demanding the best from yourself in future.

★ What Works for You: the detailed questions at the beginning of this chapter are designed to get you into the habit of constantly re-evaluating your progress and updating your view of yourself. Slimming is a process of change and once you've opened your mind to the idea of change, anything is possible. Lighten Up isn't something you do once and finish, it's just giving yourself a head start in what's going to be an ongoing programme of change and development.

★ Get What You Want: making the most of your own brainpower to ask yourself positive, motivating questions.

★ Use Your Brain: mind and body teamwork.

★ Manage yourself: staying on track with your slimming goals.

★ Be self-reliant: coping on your own and under pressure.

★ The Diet of Champions: strengthening your belief in yourself.

★ The Lighten Up Diary for Life.

WHAT WORKS FOR YOU?

 What's the difference that's made a difference? What's worked for you so far? Could you do more of it? Do you still have some ideas you haven't tried yet?

What is your Food Profile looking like now?
★ Is it nicely balanced?   Yes No
★ Are you drinking enough water?   Yes No
★ Are you eating enough fresh fruit and vegetables? Yes No
★ What changes have you made so far?

....

★ What could you do to improve it?

....

Did you track your energy levels on the graphs? Yes No
★ Is your energy affected by what you eat?   Yes No
★ By relaxation?   Yes No
★ By exercise?   Yes No
★ What else affects your energy levels?

....

....

Are you aware of any negative feelings that you still have which are associated with food?   Yes No
★ Do you have any anxiety about eating?   Yes No
★ Do you have any uncontrollable cravings
   around food?   Yes No
★ Have any of those feelings changed over the
   past eight weeks?   Yes No
★ If you answered yes to any of the above, what
   could you do to help cope with these feelings
   or change them?

....

....

Do you now have any more positive feelings towards food?   Yes   No
★ More pleasure in actually eating?   Yes   No
★ Enjoyment of cooking and shopping?   Yes   No
★ Have those feelings changed over the past
  eight weeks?   Yes   No
★ What could you do to get even more pleasure
  from the food you eat?

  ....

How are you getting on with the Hunger Scale?
★ Do you usually eat at more than 6?   Yes   No
★ Do you often eat at less than 5?   Yes   No
★ How often do you check the
  Hunger Scale?   Sometimes   Mostly   Always
★ What more could you do to make the Hunger
  Scale a totally automatic process?

  ....

Is Think Before You Eat working for you?   Yes   No
★ Do you always Think Before You Eat?   Yes   No
★ Do you mostly Think Before You Eat?   Yes   No
★ Do you usually get the right
  answer?   Sometimes   Mostly   Always
★ What more could you do to make Think Before
  You Eat faster and more instinctive?

  ....

Are you Thinking Before You Shop?   Yes   No
★ Do you plan your basic meals for the week?   Yes   No
★ Have you stocked up a store-cupboard so that you
  can always prepare something simple instead of
  having to resort to a takeaway?   Yes   No
★ Do you carry a couple of snacks – like fruit,
  for example – and some water with you, just
  in case you get stuck somewhere and you're
  hungry?   Sometimes   Mostly   Always

Has the Fat Jar helped you to get more activity into your daily life? Yes No

★ How many coins (Fat Burning Pills) do you put in every day? ....

★ How many coins would you like to put in every day? ....

★ Would you like to use the Fat Jar more often, and, if so, what could you do to make that happen? Yes No

....

Have you got some regular Feel Good Fitness exercise in your life now? Yes No

★ Are you doing this at least four times a week now? Yes No

★ How many times a week would you like to be doing it? ....

★ Do you enjoy it? Sometimes Mostly Always

★ Have you found the right form of exercise for you yet? Yes No

★ What else could you do to make this easier and more fun?

....

Are you building any of the relaxation techniques into your life? Yes No

★ Could some of these relaxation techniques underpin your general attitude to life so that you stay calmer than you used to? Yes No

★ Can you use any of the relaxation techniques as emergency measures to help you cope when you are under pressure? Yes No

★ Do you always remember to do them? Sometimes Mostly Always

★ What other forms of relaxation could you use instead of responding to stress by overeating?

....

....

How many of the ideas and exercises you've experimented with over the past weeks do you think you will keep? ....

Will you continue using the following exercises frequently.

★ Changing Your Association With Food   Yes   No
★ Sound Effects   Yes   No
★ Breathing techniques   Yes   No
★ Affirmations   Yes   No
★ Visualisation (the Movie and the Open Door)   Yes   No

Have your beliefs about yourself changed?   Yes   No

★ Do you believe you are becoming slimmer, fitter and healthier?   Yes   No
★ What are you doing to support your beliefs?

....

★ What else could you do to make your belief in yourself much stronger?

....

Have you been keeping in touch with your original slimming goal since you started this programme?   Yes   No

★ Write your slimming goal down again and notice whether it has changed.

....

★ Are you setting daily outcomes to keep you on the track of that goal?   Yes   No
★ Write down your outcomes for today.

....

....

Are you making more of a meal of eating?   Yes   No

★ Are you eating some of your meals without doing anything else at the same time?   Yes   No
★ Have you slowed down your eating?   Yes   No

★ Do you pause between mouthfuls?　　　　Yes　No
★ If you have changed your eating style, has it
　made any difference to your enjoyment of food?　Yes　No

Are you still being triggered to eat for reasons other than hunger?　　Yes　No

★ When that happens, do you go
　ahead and eat?　　Always　Mostly　Sometimes　Never
★ When you *don't* go ahead and eat, what do
　you now do instead?

....

....

Are you turning failures into feedback?　　Yes　No

★ Can you think of a time when you lapsed or
　failed during the Eight-week Programme?　　Yes　No
★ Did you learn anything from that experience
　at the time?　　Yes　No
★ Looking back on that experience now, can you
　see anything that you missed at the time?　　Yes　No
★ What could you learn now from that experience?

....

What's new in your life since you started the Eight-week Programme?

★ Activities?　　Yes　No
★ Forms of exercise?　　Yes　No
★ Types of food?　　Sometimes　Mostly　Always
★ What change in your eating or behaviour patterns
　has taken you furthest outside your comfort zone?

....

★ What change in your eating or behaviour
　patterns has been most useful in moving you
　towards your slimming goal?

....

....

Have your drinking patterns changed?   Yes   No
- ★ More water?   Yes   No
- ★ Less alcohol?   Yes   No
- ★ Less caffeine (tea, coffee, Coca-Cola)?   Yes   No
- ★ Fewer sweetened drinks?   Yes   No

Have you made friends with yourself yet?   Yes   No
- ★ When you picture yourself, is it a positive image?   Yes   No
- ★ Do you feel more respectful of your body?   Yes   No
- ★ Are you giving yourself credit for your successes and achievements?   Yes   No
- ★ Do you talk to yourself in a more positive way?   Yes   No
- ★ What new strategies have you developed for coping with stress?

....

Do you still own a pair of scales?   Yes   No
- ★ Do you want to weigh yourself?   Yes   No
- ★ Do you want to check your measurements?   Yes   No
- ★ Does it matter?   Yes   No
- ★ If it does matter, just do it. Then don't do it again for another eight weeks.

GETTING WHAT YOU WANT

It's a good idea to get into the habit of reviewing your progress by constantly asking yourself questions rather than by sneaking into the bathroom and hopping on the scales. We don't ask ourselves enough questions. In fact, we often don't like it when somebody else asks us questions. People get quite cross about it on the eight-week course sometimes. 'I'm always going to have a weight problem,' somebody said the other day.

'How do you know that?'

She looked surprised. 'I always have had one.'

'But you haven't lived your future yet, have you?'

'I sometimes wish you'd give us a diet sheet and be done with it,' she said.

Well, of course, that seems like the easy option. But apart from the fact that, as we know by now, diets don't work, crawling back into your comfort zone and counting calories for a few weeks will interrupt the long-term changes that are leading you towards being permanently slimmer. It just reinforces the old pattern of dieting and gaining weight, and losing heart over and over again. If we gave you a diet sheet and told you to turn off your brain and do it, two things would happen: your self-esteem would go down and your weight would go up – obviously neither of them results we want to see even in the short term.

So once you've finished this course and we're not here to keep challenging you every week it's going to be up to you to challenge yourself. The best way to do that is by asking yourself good questions. Why? Because questions are much more useful than statements. As soon as you turn a statement into a question it's no longer a certainty. The statement could change and you could change. Questions create choices.

SOME GOOD QUESTIONS

If you want to load the dice in your favour and go for positive changes rather than negative ones, all you have to do is play around with the wording. You know what's coming now, don't you? We've been banging on about the importance of wording your goals, outcomes, affirmations and statements positively since Chapter One. And the same rule applies to questions. The questions you ask yourself have a major effect on the quality of your life.

People who are overweight ask questions like 'Why am I so fat?' and they often get answers like 'Because you eat so much' or 'Because you have no self-control'. If you ask yourself negative questions your brain will come up with negative answers. If you constantly run this depressing stuff in your mind, you're going to make yourself feel bad. Saying 'Why does this always happen to me?' won't empower you. It will make you focus on what isn't working in your life. It will depress you and it isn't going to spur you into positive, affirmative action.

DO THIS NOW Answer these questions in your mind as you read through them.

★ Do you have certain emotions on a daily basis that you don't like?
★ What are they?
★ Did you know that these emotions grow out of the questions you ask yourself? Can you think of what any of these questions might be?

Just suppose, instead of asking questions like 'Why can't I ever stick with a diet?' you were to ask ones like:

★ 'What's great about what I am doing?'
★ 'How can I become slimmer right now'?
★ 'What can I do that will start me on the road to becoming slimmer?'
★ 'What do I need to do to make sure that I have a great day?'

Positive questions get positive answers. You could go a step further and ask:

★ 'How can I become slimmer and enjoy the process?'
★ 'How good am I going to feel when I've been for a walk and I'm soaking in a hot bath?'
★ 'What are the benefits I get from being slimmer, fitter and healthier?'
★ 'How does eating a healthy balanced diet make me feel good?'

What a concept! Your brain will happily search for a quality answer because if you give it half a chance it will do anything to avoid pain and gain pleasure. What you focus on is what you get. By asking yourself empowering questions, you begin to create positive possibilities.

USING YOUR BRAIN

If you want to be slim, you're going to have to make more use of your body. However, if you work on your body without engaging your mind first you'll be doomed to failure. So, as usual, we are starting from the head down.

Half the people who buy a computer only use a quarter of its capacity. Most people who buy sports cars don't drive them to within more than three-quarters of their potential performance.

YOU'RE AMAZING

We were all *born* with a computer more powerful than anything we could buy and we use much less than a quarter of it most of the time. We don't use our brains enough and we often neglect our bodies too. Every one of us is a more sophisticated and highly tuned machine than the highest-performance cars on the road – and we don't even bother to look after ourselves properly or use the best fuel.

Of course, you can't actually turn your brain off; it's soaking up information like a sponge all the time. But without direction from you, it will just absorb the problems you focus your attention on (like your weight). Think of someone who's a role model for you. It might be somebody richer or more successful, somebody with a bigger car or a lower golf handicap. Or it might just be somebody slimmer. What's the difference between you and your role model? Is it really just the luck of the genetic lottery, or does it have more to do with your beliefs about yourself?

It doesn't matter whether it's hip size or happiness that's important to you. The winners in life are the people who have learned to use their minds and bodies on full power all the time and not to skimp on the maintenance. Of course, we don't come with a user's manual; we have to write our own. Which is the Lighten Up Diary.

You can waste brainpower by running low-grade software all the time. If the only screen saver you have is a line that floats around saying 'I must lose some weight', this may be a sign that your software needs upgrading. Install a positive message and you're much more likely to get a positive result.

If you must ask yourself leading questions, at least make sure they are leading you in the right direction. Asking yourself encouraging questions will help you to become more resourceful and empowered. We all need some encouragement – and the surest way to get it is to build it into our own brains.

GETTING IT TOGETHER

THE DREAM TEAM

Your body and your brain are the ultimate dream team. The visualisation and goal-setting exercises we've been practising over the past few weeks have been aimed at getting you to engage your mind before you start making drastic physical changes.

DO IT YOURSELF

At the end of the eight-week course, somebody always says rather anxiously: 'All this stuff is fine when we're coming for a motivational top-up every week. But what's going to happen next week and the week after when we're back to coping on our own?'

The answer is always the same – if you want to be slim for the rest of your life, the only way is to **do it yourself**. If you take on board even a few of the ideas in this book, you will see some amazing changes (make sure you keep the Hunger Scale and Think Before You Eat). If you continue to visualise, set yourself goals and include more exercise in your life, you will be unstoppable.

COPING UNDER PRESSURE

Some of you might feel vulnerable just now. You're worried that next time there's a crisis at work, or at home, or your friends give you a hard time, or you get a cold, or go on holiday, or have one of 'those' birthdays, you'll give in to a few beers and a curry, feel rough in the morning and label yourself a failure.

Just remember that you have the power to turn things round.

GETTING IN A RIGHT STATE

It's not actually the crisis, or the relationship or the illness, or the celebration that causes the problem – it's your reaction to them. To some people a party is an excuse to dance and flirt, for others it's a calorie swamp they could drown in. It all depends on your point of view.

If you know how to worry, you also know how to motivate yourself. The process is exactly the same. The difference is that worry is a form of self-harassment that doesn't do you any good. Instead, why not use all that mental energy to put yourself in a strong, confident, dynamic frame of mind?

DO THIS NOW Is there anything in the near future that might challenge your progress towards becoming slimmer, fitter and healthier?

....

What could you do, before then, to put yourself in the best possible state to be able to cope?

....
....
....

What did you come up with? Relaxation? More Affirmations? Exercise? Sabotage Avoidance?

Here's a hint – if it's a specific event that's worrying you, do the Open Door exercise a couple of times in the hours leading up to it and then rehearse the actual event. Imagine yourself walking into that situation strong, confident and successful. Imagine you are an athlete about to compete in a race; before you go on to the track you will run the race in your mind, over and over again. And you will always win.

STAY ON TRACK

Success at slimming, sport or anything else has more to do with what you do than with where you start. So no matter how much you weigh now and how stressful your life may be, if you single-mindedly focus on the Lighten Up programme you will succeed.

Just recently, Sally Gunnell came along to talk to a new group of Lighten Up franchisees. One of them said to her, 'It must be hard for you to understand how desperate somebody feels when they've been overweight for years and they can't even run upstairs without feeling breathless. After all, you've always been slim and super-fit, haven't you?'

Then Sally told them the story of the World Championships 400 Metre Hurdle final. She caught a cold before the race, and in normal circumstances she'd have stopped training for a bit and given her body time to recover. But this time it was different. Literally facing the chance of a lifetime, she didn't even allow the possibility of pulling out to enter her mind. It was doubly difficult, of course, because not only did she have to race, she had to look as if she was on peak form so that her fellow competitors didn't realise she might be vulnerable. For days before the race she competed and won, over and over and over again – in her mind. On the day of the race she knew she was being watched by billions of people, at the stadium and on TV around the world. She recalls being aware of negative thoughts, but she shut them out and focused on her only possible outcome for the day: winning the gold medal.

The difference that will make the difference for you is the same as the one that did it for Sally. You have the power and the information you need to control your body and mind. So next time your train is late, your report is overdue or the boiler breaks down, don't make matters worse by beating yourself up and buying Dime bars on the way home. Just fix the problem and move on.

If you believe in yourself, as Sally did, you will succeed.

THE POWER OF BELIEF

The Lighten Up programme emphasises self-belief because it's the foundation of your success. When it comes to coping with stress, pressures of life, other people and the temptation of a plate of chips, there's simply no substitute for a firm foundation of belief in yourself. Many people who come to Lighten Up have no idea just how strong and potentially successful they are. They have been taught, like most of us, not to dwell on their own successes but instead to look for the areas they needed to improve. It's the old story – they were focusing on failure.

In Week One we asked you to remember times you've been a role model for yourself – when you made a decision, no matter how small and then went right ahead and achieved it. And in Chapter Thirteen you made a movie, based on three snapshots of yourself achieving your goals. For the rest of your life we want you to continue to use yourself as a resource in that way. Of course, it's also a good idea to have as many role models as you can – but when you see somebody doing something well, don't ask why they are so fortunate, ask how they did it. And because you can learn so much more from what you already do well, and by accessing your own strengths, it's worth going over this exercise one more time.

 Go back again and think of some more examples from your past when:

★ you performed a task well;
★ you were praised for a job well done;
★ you overcame obstacles;
★ you gave 100 per cent to what you were doing;
★ you did something you'd have admired in somebody else;
★ you learned a new skill (no matter how small);
★ you succeeded in one of the challenges we've set you over the past seven weeks.

Go for quantity first, then size. It doesn't matter how small you start, as long as you start somewhere – it can be anything from changing your first plug to knitting a sweater or being promoted to the top of a multinational corporation. Aim to get about 150 of these positive experiences down on paper.

DEVELOPING STRONG USEFUL BELIEFS

Now you're going to take that list and use it, to make an internal movie. Rather like the film you made in Chapter Thirteen.

★ Pick a few positive experiences from the list and arrange them into one movie – a documentary where you are the director.

★ Watch the film in your mind from beginning to end several times. See yourself on the imaginary screen from the outside, as if you were a someone you didn't know.

★ On the basis of what you see in the movie, what can you truthfully say about the person featured in it? For example:

- 'He's determined to stick with it, even when things aren't going very well.'
- 'She's got a tremendous amount of focus and concentration on what she wants.'
- 'He's very dedicated to learning and improving.'

★ Now watch the film again and this time do it from the inside as if you are actually experiencing the events as they happen. See the things you saw, hear the things you heard and feel the things you felt. The only difference is that everything happens in the order you, as director, want to put them in, rather than the way they happened in life.

Run through the film to the end and when you've finished, make that comment to yourself again, the one you made at the third step. But this time make it an 'I' statement: 'I really stick with it, even when things aren't going very well.' Say it with conviction; say it like you mean it.

THE DIET OF CHAMPIONS

So here you are, at the end of the Lighten Up Eight-week Course. And here, at last, is the diet you've been waiting for:

Desire your Outcome
Imagine achieving it
Expect to succeed
Take Time to reach your goal

DESIRE

Like most successful sportspeople, Sally Gunnell's desire to be a winner was strong enough to drive her to succeed, whatever the odds against her. It's important to ask yourself how much you really want to achieve your goal. Sure, you'd like to be fitter – wouldn't everybody? But do you want it enough to give up going to the pub three nights a week? Do you want it enough to give up your lunch hour three times a week? Do you want it enough to get out of bed an hour earlier in the mornings?

What are you *actually* prepared to do to get it?

Remember you're a pleasure seeker, we all are. So if you're going to give up something you love, like curling up with some chocolate and a video, your desire to be slimmer and fitter will need to be very powerful. So be realistic about it. Take a cool look at what it is you want and ask yourself how passionately you want it. If you don't want it passionately enough, then raise your motivation levels (take a look back at Chapter Eight). When the idea of being slimmer and fitter becomes more compelling than watching superheroes from the sofa, you stand a good chance of long-term success.

IMAGINATION

Your imagination is the most powerful tool you possess. You can use it to make anything possible. Once you have that picture of your future slimmer, fitter, richer, happier self firmly fixed in your line of vision, you'll find your brain will start supplying you with appropriate sounds and feelings too. And once you're mentally test-driving your new self, you'll probably find yourself living the way your new self would want to live. Maybe your new slimmer self doesn't eat Mars bars; maybe your new slimmer self takes more exercise; maybe your new slimmer self will be kinder and more encouraging when you start making those changes . . .

Recent research using biofeedback machines shows that resting athletes who vividly imagine they are in competition will experience changes in their heart rate, blood pressure and body temperature – just as if they are actually out on the track. So athletes (and everybody else) can feel like winners whenever and wherever they want.

Prince Naseem is often asked how he predicts his winning rounds. He tells reporters that for weeks before a fight he spends every spare moment imagining himself fighting his opponent. He plays the experience in full colour, with surround sound. It's a movie he runs in his head with himself as director and producer as well as the star. Athletes like Naseem often get a déjà vu effect on the day of the event – they've already tasted victory in their minds (and bodies) so many times. The key is to practise until your images become second nature and seem absolutely real.

EXPECTATION

Every time you use your imagination like this, you are building a powerful belief in yourself and you can begin to expect results. Very often, people who make New Year resolutions hope they will succeed. Hope leaves things to chance. Can you imagine Prince Naseem walking into the ring, looking at his opponent and thinking 'I don't like the look of him . . . I hope he's not as fast as he looks . . . I'd better try a bit of positive thinking'?

The British are great believers in not expecting too much. In fact, it's one of those pieces of advice that elderly relatives and depressed parents hand out to children. Why didn't we ever answer back and say 'Why not? Aren't I worth it?'

If you were raised on this theory that low expectations lead to contentment, you may need to upgrade your expectations a bit and you may find these suggestions about how you talk to yourself quite useful. Instead of trying, hoping and wishing, you must change your behaviour in the future, use the present tense and act like it's already happening.

TIME

If you want to be the best you've ever been, give yourself time – all the time you need. You may be unfit and out of shape but you didn't get that way overnight. And you won't get back in shape overnight either – whatever the latest wonder diet says. All that drastic weight loss does is make you thinner and less fit – you'll be losing water and muscle instead of fat. And that's not healthy – or permanent. This may be the age of instant everything, but your mind and body are the exceptions because, unlike most instant things, you aren't manmade. You evolved very slowly and you have the power to change your own mind and body – at the pace that's right for you, not the pace that a diet or exercise programme dictates.

If you've been inactive and eating junk for years, your body and mind will protest if you try to change. And if you ever had a blueprint for the way you were meant to be, you probably over-wrote it a long time ago.

So, are you ready to break through the discomfort barrier and make some life-enhancing changes? The first step is to give yourself time. After all, if you're out of shape, you didn't get that way overnight. Take as much time as you need to reverse the process, slowly and comfortably. That way the changes are more likely to be permanent.

 Write this down in your Diary, print it on a card and put it in your wallet, stick it on your mirror or turn it into your screen saver.

Desire your Outcome
Imagine achieving it
Expect to succeed
Take **T**ime to reach your goal

We've found this over the years, to be the greatest little reminder to keep people focused on achieving the outcomes and goals they set themselves.

THE LIGHTEN UP DIARY FOR LIFE

Continue to keep your Diary and fill in your Food Profile for the next four weeks, recording what seems important to you. After four weeks you probably won't need the Profile any more, don't spend the rest of your life writing down what you eat and drink

– just enjoy it. As for the Diary itself, that will probably either stop or evolve. It can be a great way to get personal and emotional feedback, and stay in control of your life.

CENSORSHIP

The reasons for writing the Diary become very clear at this stage as you start to do it for yourself – rather than because somebody's telling you to. You may find, as a lot of people do, that the Diary keeps you on track. Just be sure to censor it for negativity. That doesn't mean you shouldn't write down the negative stuff. Of course you'll have lapses and bad days, and you need to make a note of them so that you can look back a couple of weeks later and see how insignificant they were. That's always a very encouraging thing to do.

Just as we're always telling you to give yourself positive messages, we also suggest you write more positive things in your Diary. There are lots of reasons for keeping the Diary but one of the most important ones is to make sure that the software you're running in your brain is positive, constructive and helpful.

Our natural inclination to dwell on what's not working tends to come out a lot in diaries. So make a note of the negatives and keep an eye on trends, but make sure you write down the good stuff so you can tell how *well* you're doing. Then you can congratulate yourself and take heart from it and be your own role model more often. Write down what you've *learned* from the things that go wrong – that's much more important than recording the actual disasters. Write down the things you've achieved, how you've felt about them and the progress you're making towards your goal. When you reach that goal, set yourself a new one. Positive changes never let you rest. Once you're hooked on change you'll find you have to keep going. It's an addiction of the best kind.

Give your mind and body time to settle into a new way of living. It's time to consider new ways of seeing things, new attitudes and new methods of self-management.

Finally, and very important, give yourself credit when you change a habit that has been limiting your life for years. And give yourself a pat on the back each time you recognise the difference between being hungry and thirsty, or just plain bored and fed up.

CHALLENGES

This week you get all the exercises in the book as your Challenges. Of course you can cherry pick, but give the ones that didn't work first time a second (or third) chance.

★ Make regular Feel Good Fitness and Fat Jar Fitness – Fat Burning Pills – a part of your life for the rest of your life. Fat Jar Fitness is the most important: if you start to lead a more active life you're less likely to lapse because it will be part of what you do every day. But if you can also make four or more sessions of Feel Good Fitness a part of your life, you will find it works wonders for your state of mind as well as your size and shape. It doesn't have to be a chore – it doesn't have to mean going to the gym and working out. There are so many things you could do, from dancing to yoga, pilates or swimming. All of them will make you feel good and none of them need take more than a couple hours out of your day (at most). If you just opt for a half-hour exercise session at home it could be just an hour – including the shower!

★ Relax more often as you learn to respond to stress in other ways than reaching for the HobNobs. Experiment with the relaxation techniques we've suggested and research some more of your own until you find the ones that work for you. Use the chilling-out technique and breathing exercises at every opportunity.

★ Continue to feel good for no good reason. Come to think of it, any reason to feel good is a good reason, isn't it?

★ Keep using the Hunger Scale until you are doing it automatically.

★ Carry on Thinking Before You Eat until it's programmed into your eating patterns. It's like a shield you can carry for the rest of your life that will protect you from eating the wrong things.

★ Daydream on. This is the fun bit. Whenever you get disheartened, or you can't cope with working out your Hunger Scale, try a bit of daydreaming with intent. Catching a glimpse of the future you as you want to be is very energising.

★ Make sure you get plenty of health food for your mind as well as your body – focus on positive questions and thoughts.

★ Design yourself a plan of action for the next month.

★ Make a contract with yourself to follow the plan.

★ If and when you have a lapse, follow the Success Formula in Week Four.

★ Write on a piece of card, two or three things that would bring you closer to your goal if you did them every day. They are the legs that support your belief in yourself as a slim person. They can also double up as your outcomes for the day but review them regularly because these things change and evolve, just as you do.

★ On another piece of card or in your Lighten Up Diary, on your laptop or in your Filofax, write down a list of emergency quick fixes that you can use if you have a problem. The Sound Effects exercise, the Changing Association With Food exercise, some displacement activities and some social pressure strategies perhaps – just some little reminders of things that might help if times get tough.

★ If you are looking for inspiration to cook healthy meals, turn to the back of the book and experiment with some of the recipes. They aren't necessarily meant to be followed to the letter. You can add your own variations to all of them.

THE LIGHTEN UP CHECKLIST

It's up to you now to draw up a checklist that might see you through the next few days or weeks (or years). Or you might feel that you're past the checklist stage and that you can go freestyle.

	M	T	W	T	F	S	S

My goal for the future is:

....

....

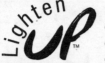 Write a letter to yourself about how you achieved your goal, seal it up, address the envelope, stamp it and write on the back the date you would like to receive it. Put it inside another envelope and send it to us at Lighten Up. The address is on page 419.

We will post it back to you on the date you've chosen.

PART

3

THE LIGHTEN UP FOOD PROFILE[1]

Warning: before changing your diet, always take advice from your doctor. Some individuals may have adverse reactions to foods which don't seem to affect others. It is well known that some people are allergic to nuts but it's also possible to react badly to almost any food including uncooked vegetables. This is very unusual, but it can happen. If you are going to eat anything you haven't tried before, or you are trying something raw that you've always eaten cooked, please be cautious.

As we explained in Week Four, the Food Profile is a visual guide to help you see how healthy or unhealthy your eating patterns are at the moment. Fill in everything you eat and drink in the appropriate circle, starting from the centre and moving out. If you run out of circles, draw another one round the outside.

During the second four weeks of the Lighten Up programme, most people notice a significant shift in emphasis from the Foods to Limit circle towards the Foods to Focus On. You should

---

1 The Lighten Up Food Profile was developed from an original idea by Justin Roberts.

FOODS TO FOCUS ON

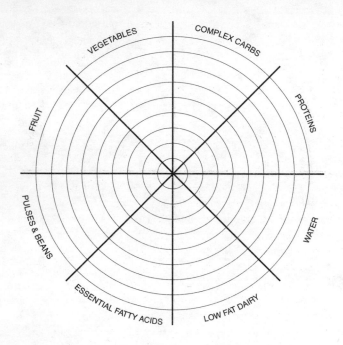

Fruit
Vegetables
Complex Carbohydrates: bread, cereals, grains, potatoes
Proteins: lean meat, fish and poultry
Pulses, Lentils and Beans
Essential Fatty Acids
Low-fat Dairy
Water

You should be drinking around two litres of water and eating at least five servings of fruit or vegetables every day. We don't make specific recommendations for any of the other categories – it depends on you and your lifestyle.

FOODS TO LIMIT

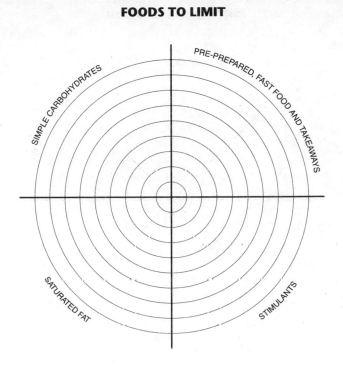

Simple Carbohydrates: sugar
Pre-prepared, Fast Food and Takeaways
Saturated Fat: red meat and full-fat dairy
Stimulants: tea, coffee, alcohol, plain chocolate

There are no daily minimum requirements for any of these!
If you decide you can live without any of them, that's great.

aim, eventually, to be eating most of your daily requirements from the left-hand circle.

Put a cross for every portion of food you eat in the appropriate circle. If it's fast food or a takeaway (and that includes any pre-prepared meals you just buy and stick in the microwave), here are some guidelines:

★ Don't try to split it up into carbohydrate or protein, just put one cross in the fast-food section of Foods to Limit.

★ If you are having just a bag of chips or a burger or a kebab, one cross is fine but if you're going the whole hog and having large fries and a Big Mac as well, put two crosses.

★ The Coca-Cola and apple pie you might order at the same time will be two separate crosses in the simple carbohydrates section.

★ We haven't included restaurant meals as fast foods because many restaurants do have healthier options and you can be selective with the menu. You can always opt for salads (and ask for it to be served without dressing), vegetables, or grilled fish and avoid the chips and puddings. Takeaways aren't usually that flexible and they are almost always higher in fat anyway. So if you're eating at a place which offers you a reasonable choice, just split up the components as if you were eating at home (remember, it doesn't have to be exact, just roughly estimate what categories most of the food would fall into).

On pages 322–5 are two examples of how a Food Profile might be filled in. You'll notice that one person has chosen healthier options than the other – but even she wasn't perfect.

FILLING IN THE FOOD PROFILE

The categories on the Profile don't correspond to particular nutritional food groups – we've just set them up in a way that should make it easy to enter what you've eaten.

Some foods may seem difficult to categorise at first. Digestive biscuits, for example, go into the simple carbohydrate (sugar) section although they also contain some complex carbohydrate (wheat flour) and saturated fat. They're simple carbohydrates because sugar is their main ingredient, like most biscuits, cakes and puddings, and the saturated fat they contain would have to go into the Foods to Limit section anyway. And if that doesn't convince you, even the complex carbohydrate they contain is mostly very refined and not very good for you. So, we're afraid all your sweet treats and desserts have to be entered as simple carbohydrates.

You're probably wondering how much to divide your foods between different categories and the answer is to keep it as simple as you can. You can separate out a sandwich and its filling, and you might want to make a note of the sugar in your tea. But by and large, just put everything down in whichever category seems the most obvious. Over a whole day, or a week, your Food Profile will be as accurate as you need it to be.

If you really get stuck on something like salmon which contains protein *and* essential fatty acids, then put a cross in both sections of the Food Profile if you like – it doesn't matter much when foods are split between the good food groups because all your crosses are accumulating in the healthy circle anyway. It's more of a nuisance if you eat something that's split between Foods to Focus On and Foods to Limit, but it's best to be honest and put your two crosses in the appropriate sections anyway. For example, if you have a bowl of strawberries and put sugar all over them, put your cross in both fruit and simple carbohydrates (sugar).

The food lists at the end of this chapter will help you to begin with, but it won't be long before you find you don't need to keep referring to them.

Now, before you start filling in your Food Profile for today, here are some basic hints about healthy eating.

Helpful hints

★ Whenever possible, choose fresh foods with no additives, preservatives, E numbers or added sugar and eat some of them raw. If you aren't sure what something's made of, check the label.

HEALTHY FOOD PROFILE

Breakfast
Unsweetened muesli (complex carbohydrate)
Skimmed milk (low-fat dairy)
Orange juice (fruit)
Banana (fruit)

Lunch
Vegetable soup (vegetables)
Wholemeal bread (complex carbohydrate)

Snacks
Black coffee (stimulant)
Apple (fruit)
½ Mango (fruit)
Strawberries (fruit)

2½ litres Water

Dinner
Salmon (protein)
New Potatoes (complex carbohydrate)
Peas (vegetable)
Apricot Tart (simple carbohydrate)
Cream (saturated fat)
Glass of Wine (stimulant)

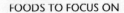

FOODS TO FOCUS ON

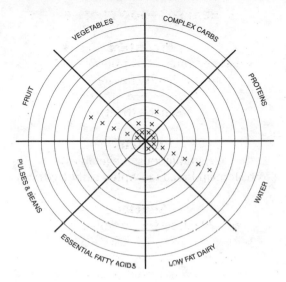

FOODS TO LIMIT

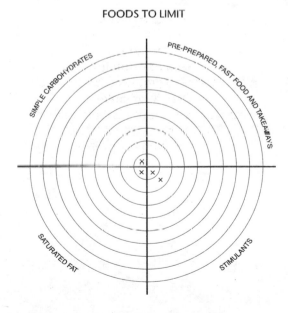

NOT SO HEALTHY FOOD PROFILE

Breakfast
2 grilled tomatoes (vegetables)
Fried bread (complex carbohydrate + saturated fat)
2 sausages (saturated fat)
White toast, butter, jam
(complex carbohydrate + simple carbohydrate +
saturated fat)
2 mugs tea with sugar
(stimulants x 2 + simple carbohydrates x 2)

Snack
Apple (fruit)
Can Lilt (simple carbohydrate)

Lunch
Cheese and Pickle sandwiches on white
(complex carbohydrate + saturated fat)
Penguin (simple carbohydrate)
Can Coke (simple carbohydrate)

Snacks
2 mugs tea with sugar
(stimulants + simple carbohydrates)
2 digestives (simple carbohydrates)
Peanuts (saturated fats)

Dinner
Pepperoni Pizza (pre-prepared fast food)
Salad (vegetable)
Unsweetened fruit salad (fruit)
2 pints lager (stimulant)
Double brandy (stimulant)

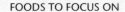

FOODS TO FOCUS ON

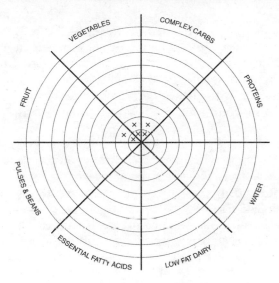

FOODS TO LIMIT

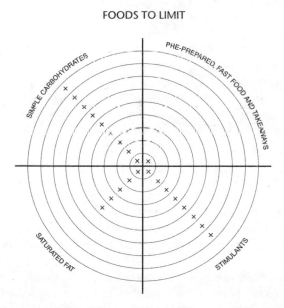

★ Complex carbohydrates are better for you when they're unrefined because they have more nutritional value and they're less likely to contain hidden sugar – it's surprising how much sugar is added to processed food. Some of the basic complex carbohydrate types of food which we regard as staples (like white bread, for example) contain a lot of hidden sugar, so choose wholemeal bread and include more brown rice, wholewheat pasta and other unrefined sources of carbohydrate as often as you can. (See the lists in this chapter for more ideas.)

★ Vegetables are extremely important so we haven't split them up into different categories. As long as you don't add sugar or overcook them, they are all good for you. Be aware, however, that some of them contain much more carbohydrate than others. For this reason we've actually put potatoes in the complex carbohydrate category instead of listing them with the other vegetables (yes, there are lots of other starchy vegetables – like parsnips, sweetcorn and peas – but we don't tend to eat them as often as we eat potatoes).

★ Fruit is also a vital part of healthy eating but some fruits are sweeter than others (more about this later). Eat your fruit before it gets overripe and don't add sugar to it.

★ Cut down on refined sugars, salt and caffeine. They play havoc with the body, confusing and interrupting the natural running order.

★ Drink plain water rather than fizzy water, which is acidic, or flavoured water, which may contain chemicals, sweeteners and sugar.

★ Give yourself time and space to eat and enjoy your meals so your digestion can get the maximum nutritional value from what you eat.

★ Eat less red meat and deep-fried food so you don't overload your body with saturated fat, which is very easy to store and carry around with you. When you choose red meat instead of chicken or rabbit, you are getting high quality protein but a lot of saturated fat as well which is why red meat and saturated fat go in the same section on the Foods to Limit circle.

★ Don't get fanatical about fat. You need to eat some every day, so whenever possible choose polyunsaturated or monounsaturated fats rather than saturated ones (see lists which follow). Nuts and seeds are a good source of the right kind of fat and they also contain energy, protein, vitamins and minerals, but check the list to see which are the good ones – some of them also contain saturated fat.

★ Be creative, try different grains, fruits and vegetables, and experiment with new recipes.

★ Vegetarians can substitute beans, lentils, tofu or soya for meat. It's a good idea to eat as many different kinds of protein as possible.

★ Add flavour to your cooking with herbs and spices rather than extra salt or fat.

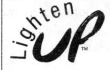

The more variety you include in your diet the healthier you will be.

THE FOOD LISTS

None of these lists is comprehensive, but they should give you an idea of what kinds of food fit into each category. If the food you want to eat isn't on the list, don't panic. You'll have a good idea of where it fits in by the time you've finished this chapter.

Foods to Focus On

FRUIT

One Serving:
1 large fruit (apple, orange, peach)
Small glass of unsweetened juice
1 cup of berries or pineapple
2 handfuls[2] of cherries or grapes
2 handfuls of raisins

2 Handfuls vary according to the size of their owner, which makes them good food measures.

Fruit plays an important part in a balanced diet. Many fruits contain lots of vitamins (particularly A and C), fibre and minerals. Fruit is low in fat and is handy for snacks. Yes, it does contain sugar, but the sugar isn't empty calories like candy floss – and fruit is so rich in other nutrients that you should make it an important part of your diet. Some of the most easily available are:

Apples
Apricots
Bananas
Berries
Cherries
Dried fruit (not processed or sugared)
Figs
Grapefruit
Grapes
Kiwis
Lemons
Mangoes
Melons
Nectarines
Oranges
Peaches
Pears
Pineapples
Plums
Rhubarb

VEGETABLES

One Serving:
1 cup of raw or cooked vegetables

Vegetables should also be a major part of a healthy, balanced diet. They are an excellent form of carbohydrate and contain lots of vitamins (especially A and C) and minerals (iron and magnesium). They are a valuable source of antioxidants, which help protect against degenerative diseases, including cancer and heart disease, and contain soluble and insoluble fibre, which help to lower blood cholesterol levels. They are low in calories and fat, and most of them are low in sugar too, so they are generally good news for people wanting to lose weight.

It's best to undercook them and you can eat some of them without cooking them at all. Obviously certain vegetables (turnips and asparagus, for example) are inedible if they aren't cooked, so always check if you're eating something raw for the first time. Occasionally someone can react badly to an under-cooked vegetable and there are some vegetables (like kidney beans) that should *always* be well cooked. If you're not sure about it, check before you eat it. Here's a selection:

Asparagus	Leeks
Aubergines	Lettuce
Avocados	Mushrooms
Beetroot	Okra
Broccoli	Onions
Brussels sprouts	Parsley
Carrots	Peas
Cauliflower	Peppers
Celery	Spinach
Courgettes	Sprouted beans
Cucumbers	Swede
Fennel	Sweetcorn
Garlic	Tomatoes
Kale	Watercress

COMPLEX CARBOHYDRATES: BREAD, POTATOES, CEREALS AND GRAINS

One Serving:
1 cup cooked grain e.g. rice
1 cup pasta or potatoes
1 cup unsweetened cereal
2 slices bread or 2 small rolls

Much of our carbohydrate tends to be eaten in the form of bread and there's an amazing variety of it to choose from. Some bread is highly refined and contains hidden sugar, so check the packaging. Breakfast cereals are another popular source of carbohydrate and vary from natural to highly processed, so check the packets to work out the proportion of sugar to carbohydrate.

Barley
Buckwheat
Bulgar
Corn
Couscous
Keniou
Millet
Oats
Pasta (usually wheat, can be other grains)
Potatoes
Rice: brown, basmati, wild, red
Rye
Spelt
Wheat

PULSES, LENTILS AND BEANS

One Serving:
1 cup beans
85g/3oz soya or tofu

Black-eye beans
Butter beans
Chickpeas
Kidney beans (must be well cooked)
Lentils (red and brown) and lentil flour
Lima beans
Soya beans & Tofu (which is made out of soya beans)
Split peas
Tofu

MEAT, FISH AND POULTRY

One Serving:
85g/3oz lean meat, poultry, fish
1 egg white

Red meat is listed under saturated fats because, although beef, lamb and pork are wonderful sources of complete protein, they tend to be very high in saturated fats. Egg yolk is high in cholesterol so we've only listed egg white in this section. We've listed all the fish here for simplicity, but be aware that you get extra benefit from oily fish as it contains large amounts of essential fatty acids as well as protein.

Chicken
Egg white
Fish
Rabbit
Turkey

All fish are an excellent source of protein; however, try to eat oily fish such as mackerel, herrings and sardines at least once a week for the essential fatty acids they contain. Tuna, swordfish, salmon, trout, halibut and turbot contain smaller amounts of the fatty acids. White fish such as cod, haddock, hake, hoki, whiting and plaice aren't good sources of EFAs (although some contain more than others) but they are still high in protein and low in saturated fats.

LOW-FAT DAIRY

One Serving:
55g/2oz low-fat cheese
1 cup non-fat milk
½ cup semi-skimmed milk
½ cup low-fat yoghurt

Dairy foods are a good source of vitamin A, vitamin D and calcium. Vitamins A and D are essential for the development and growth of skin, bones and teeth. Calcium is an essential mineral for good health.

If you are worried about eating too many dairy foods but want to be sure you are getting enough calcium, remember that tofu, made with the setting agent calcium chloride, is the richest non-dairy source of calcium.

Cottage cheese
Low-fat cheese
Low-fat milk
Low-fat yoghurt

Calcium-rich dairy substitutes:

Rice milk
Soya milk and yoghurt

WATER

If you drink a lot during the day but rarely have a glass of water on its own, ask yourself why not. Then give it a try. You could substitute some of those cups of tea or coffee and cans of Diet Coke for glasses of water and see a difference in your Food Profile balance straight away.

ESSENTIAL FATTY ACIDS (EFAs)

One Serving:
Handful of nuts
Small handful of seeds

The nuts and oils listed here contain essential fatty acids, which your body needs, and are lower in saturated fats than other nuts like peanuts and cashews. They are very good for you, but don't pig out – they take a lot of digesting. Avocados are in here as well as in the vegetable section because they are so high in essential fatty acids. Oily fish is also a great source of EFAs, as mentioned above.

Almonds
Avocados
Brazils
Hazelnuts
Pumpkin seeds
Sesame seeds
Sunflower seeds
Walnuts

Borage oil †
Flaxseed oil *
Linseed oil *
Olive oil †
Safflower oil †
Sesame oil †
Sunflower oil †

* Linseed and flaxseed are cold-pressed oils, which need to be refrigerated and shouldn't be heated, so you can't cook with them. Their structure actually changes when they are subjected to heat and they turn into a form which the body can't deal with very easily. You may decide that they are more effort than they are worth, but on the other hand they are very high in essential fatty acids and you could put them into salad dressings.

† These oils are fine for cooking, but don't heat them too much for too long. Their structure changes with heating as well, although not so drastically as linseed and flaxseed oil do.

Foods to Limit

SIMPLE CARBOHYDRATES: SUGAR

As we've already mentioned, there's more to some of the foods we've listed here than just sugar. But the proportion of healthy ingredients is generally low (raisins in a cake, for example). Many of these foods contain saturated fats and chemicals, as well as lots of sugar.

One Serving:
2 level tablespoons sugar
Small serving of dessert
Small slice of cake

Biscuits (including most muesli/oat bars)
Cakes
Cookies
Croissants
Desserts, puddings and ice-cream
Doughnuts
Flapjacks
Honey
Jam
Lemon curd
Marmalade
Pastry
Peanut butter
Sugar
Sugary drinks (Coke, Ribena, lemonade etc.)
Sweets (Mars bars etc.)
Syrup
Tinned fruit (check the labels for added sugar)
Waffles

PRE-PREPARED, FAST FOODS AND TAKEAWAYS

Don't bother trying to separate out the good ingredients from the bad – a takeaway is just a takeaway. Some will be higher in fat and additives than others, but you can safely assume that when you eat them you aren't doing yourself any favours.

You don't, however, have to give up Oriental food. Curries and stir-fries are absolutely fine if you prepare them yourself using good, fresh ingredients and limiting the saturated fat content. It's a shame that we've got so used to the commercial, fast-food versions because home cooked tastes much better.

Typical fast food & takeaways

Burgers	Indian takeaways
Chicken and chips	Kebabs
Chinese takeaways	Microwave meals
Fish and Chips	Pizzas
Full English breakfasts	Pre-prepared meals

SATURATED FATS

Most people know about the dangers of saturated fat but it's almost impossible to avoid it altogether, as it's in so many every-day foods. Don't try to cut fat out of your diet completely, simply choose EFAs over saturated fats where possible and be aware of how much saturated fat you are eating on a daily or weekly basis.

One Food Profile serving is:
4 tablespoons of cream
4 teaspoons of peanut butter
Small bag of crisps
Small portion of chips
Couple of biscuits

Beef, pork and lamb (most red meat is high in saturated fats)
Coconut milk
Cooking oils other than ones on the essential fatty acids list
Margarine and butter
Most cheeses including feta (unless reduced fat)
Peanuts
Processed meat: sausages, ham, bacon, salami etc
Whole-fat and whole-cream milk

STIMULANTS

One Serving:
1 cup of regular or ground coffee or tea
½ pint lager or beer
1 glass red or white wine

Alcohol	Plain chocolate
Coffee	Tea

Alcohol is usually classified as a depressant, but it acts as a stimulant to your adrenal system, as does caffeine, and puts a strain on your body. If you can't remember the other ways in which alcohol can slow down your slimming, take a look back at Chapter Fourteen.

What else do you need?

FOOD SUPPLEMENTS

If you eat a varied diet with most of your choices taken from the Foods to Focus On list, you should be getting all the nutrients you need. There's a lot of controversy about food supplements and current thinking is that it's best to get your vitamins and minerals direct from the food you eat rather than by taking tablets. However, if you think you are missing out on anything, either because you have a medical problem or your diet is restricted and you don't eat some of the Foods to Focus On, you should take advice from your doctor or nutritionist before deciding what supplements to take.

FIBRE

Fibre isn't one of the categories on the Food Profile because it isn't really a food. But because it's so vital to your digestive process it's very important to include it in your diet. You won't be writing it down – but be aware that you do need plenty of it. The following fruits and vegetables are especially rich in fibre.

Apples	Oranges
Bananas	Peaches
Blackberries	Pears
Broccoli	Peas
Carrots	Plain popcorn
Cauliflower	Prunes
Figs	Puffed rice
Lentils	Puffed wheat
Lightly cooked vegetables	Raspberries
Nectarines	Rye bread

Entering the lists

★ Carry your Food Profile sheet with you and fill it in as you go along.

★ If you aren't sure where to enter something, look through the lists for something similar.

★ Something that seems to be a mixture of a Food to Focus On and a Food to Limit (like a pizza with a salad, for example) should be recorded in both sections.

★ Don't forget you do have to use a bit of discretion when you enter takeaways, fast-food and pre-prepared meals – if you just have a basic burger and small fries one cross will do, but if you have a Kentucky bucketful, be fair to yourself and make it two crosses. Your Coke and ice-cream each get a separate tick in the simple carbohydrates section.

★ Wait until you've completed two or three days of the Profile before you start analysing the trends.

SOME BASICS ABOUT NUTRITION

The Food Profile is a graphic way of showing you how easy it is to ensure you're getting everything you need from your daily diet and not eating too much of the stuff your body would rather do without. And that may be all you need to help you make the changes you want to make.

But if you want a little more nutritional background information about what you eat, read on.

WHAT HAS FOOD EVER DONE FOR YOU?

Made you fat, perhaps? Made you anxious? It's easy to forget what nutrition is all about. If you were to ask a roomful of people what food meant to them, nutrition would almost certainly get fewer mentions than the other words on the following list.

Comfort	Nutrition
Danger	Obsession
Necessity	Pleasure

Food is such a basic source of pleasure and pain that we tend to overlook the fact that it also keeps us alive. And it gives us health and energy, or at least it should – eating the wrong foods can just as easily make us sick and tired. In fact, in some parts of the world nutrition is a form of medicine – a Chinese doctor will always want to know what you're eating and treatment for most things usually involves adjusting your diet. We have a long way to go in Britain before we take what we eat as seriously as the drugs the doctor prescribes. But we are finally realising that there's more to nutrition than comfort eating and getting fat.

Nutrition is a complex, fast evolving science, but the basic facts remain the same. In order to stay slim and healthy we need to eat enough from each of the six main nutrient groups on a daily basis.

EVERYBODY IS HIGH MAINTENANCE

Your body is incredibly sophisticated and its survival and functioning depend entirely on the food you put into it.

★ You renew most parts of your body every three years and all the materials for rebuilding your bones, your organs and your blood come from food.
★ The billions of individual cells that make up your body all perform different functions that keep you alive through a series of complex reactions. However, these reactions are triggered by starter chemicals which your body absorbs from your food.

YOUR INPUT

As you read this book, your body is performing thousands of tasks, which are keeping you alive. And the amazing thing is that you can make these processes more efficient by exercising regularly and eating good food.

A regular supply of nutrients helps your cells to renew themselves properly. So, given that you're eating to feed your cells and constantly renew all the tissues that make you who you are, don't you owe it to yourself to eat the best food you possibly can? And you definitely owe it to yourself not to clog up your system with empty calories and potentially harmful chemicals.

Food groups

If you fill in the Food Profile every day, you will have a good idea of how healthy and balanced your diet is. But if, in addition to this, you understand what each of the six different food groups are, it will help you make even better choices.

IMPORTANT FOOD GROUPS

To give you a clearer idea of why it's so important to have a *varied* diet we have divided the essential foods into two groups: Macronutrients and Micronutrients.

Macronutrients
Carbohydrates, *Protein* and *Fat* are the main food groups we need in large amounts. Our digestion has to work hard to turn them into a form our bodies can actually use. Carbohydrates have to be converted to glucose, fats into fatty acids and proteins into amino acids before they can actually work for us.

Micronutrients
Vitamins and *Minerals* enable our bodies to function properly, they are necessary for hormonal and nervous interactions and they regulate our metabolism. We include *Water* here as well because it is so important.

CARBOHYDRATES

Carbohydrates are a direct source of energy for the body and are divided into two types: simple and complex.

Simple Carbohydrates

Simple carbohydrates, or sugars are rapidly broken down into glucose. The fact that they hit the bloodstream so fast can cause problems (see page 342).

Complex Carbohydrates

Complex carbohydrates or starches are broken down into glucose more slowly so the body can absorb and process them more slowly and efficiently.

PROTEIN

Every single organ and body tissue is made of protein, which needs renewing constantly. Proteins are made up of amino acids which are divided into two groups: essential and non-essential.

Essential Amino Acids

There are eight essential amino acids which the body needs on a daily basis and can't manufacture. They have to come directly from the food you eat.

Non-essential Amino Acids

There are also 12 non-essential amino acids which the body can make for itself – but only if the essential ones are already present.

The best way to make sure you're getting the right kind of protein is to eat a very varied diet. People on restricted diets (including many well-known slimming plans) may not be getting enough good quality protein.

FAT

You need some fat in your diet to ensure you get the essential fatty acids your body needs, but some fats are better for you than others.

There are three types: saturated, monounsaturated and polyunsaturated.

Saturated fat

is solid at room temperature and comes mainly from meat and dairy products.

Monounsaturated Fats (olive and peanut oils).

Polyunsaturated Fats (sunflower, corn, soybean oils and fish oils).

All three have the same number of calories, but saturated fats have been linked with heart disease and other major health problems. Poly-unsaturated are the best ones to choose in order to avoid raising your cholesterol levels, although mono-unsaturated fats are better than saturated ones.

MICRONUTRIENTS

VITAMINS

Vitamins are needed for the body's normal growth and metabolism. They are organic, so you can get them from plants and animal products.

If you eat meat you're getting your vitamins second-hand from the plants the animals have eaten. It's better to get your vitamins direct, by eating the vegetables and fruit yourself – you'll get more vitamin C, for example, from an orange or even a potato than from a steak.

MINERALS

Minerals aren't organic and can't directly provide energy that your body can absorb. Instead, they keep the body functioning by enabling you to unlock the energy from the other foods you eat.

As we mentioned in Chapter 11, a lot of vital minerals get stripped out of processed and refined foods, which means the energy from these foods can't be released as they're eaten. Instead, the body has to find the minerals it needs for this process from other parts of the body. That's why, if you eat a lot of processed foods, you might have a mineral deficiency. The best way to protect yourself is to eat a varied diet and make sure it contains some of the mineral-rich foods on the next page.

WATER

Water is your most basic need after air. You'll die of thirst much faster than you'll die of hunger.

Most of your body is composed of water but not only can you not store it, you need constantly to replace it as you're losing it continually.

It's an essential internal lubricant and cleanser, it keeps your kidneys and other organs functioning and your digestive system can't function properly without it.

SUGAR AND REFINED FOODS
– A HEALTH WARNING

We've given you a lot of information about sugar in Chapter Twelve, but we want to make sure that the Lighten Up message about this simple carbohydrate is perfectly clear. When you look at food labels remember that sugar has a lot of different names. Glucose, fructose, maltose, dextrose, corn syrup, treacle and cane sugar are all types of sugar. They provide us with energy but not much else; in fact, they can actually rob our bodies of stored vitamins and minerals, which is why they're sometimes called anti nutrients.

Our bodies need two teaspoons of sugar in the bloodstream at any one time in order to function properly but, again, this is just as easily obtained from digesting complex carbohydrates like brown rice or pasta, or even from protein and fat. We have a limited amount of sugar storage in the body and, when it's full, the leftover sugar is easily converted to fat for longer-term storage.

Eating too much refined sugar is thought to be directly linked to diabetes, migraines, low immunity, skin disorders, yeast overgrowth (candida), tooth decay – and, of course, obesity. Obesity may not be classified officially as an illness, but it is increasingly associated with heart disease, cancer and many other health problems.

Although we put less sugar in our tea and on our cereal than we used to, food companies are making up for that by putting more and more of it into processed foods. According to the Department of Health, sugar consumption in Britain has risen by 31 per cent since 1980 and the average person eats between half a kilo and one kilo of it every week.[3] At least when we were spooning it on for ourselves we knew how much of the stuff we were getting. A lot of people nowadays have no idea how much sugar they are actually eating every day.

Processed and refined foods are not only sweeter (and usually higher in fat as well as lower in vitamins and minerals), they are also more easily absorbed. When you eat a complex carbohy-

3 Dr William Grant, NASA, February 1999.

drate like brown rice, for example, it takes quite a while for the various enzymes in your digestive system to break it down, so it's absorbed quite slowly. Which is exactly the way it's supposed to be. But because refined food has already been partly broken down before it even goes into your mouth, it gets absorbed into the bloodstream faster than your system is able to deal with it. You get a short energy boost from a Mars bar, but the brown rice will give you a much more sustained release of glucose into the bloodstream.

Hypoglycaemia (low blood sugar)

The problem with sugar – or simple carbohydrate – is the dramatic effect it tends to have on the body. Because it's absorbed so much faster than complex carbohydrates it can cause sudden changes in blood sugar level and that can be dangerous. Of course, that rapid but temporary 'high' we get from sugar is one of the reasons we use it to perk us up when we're feeling down. It's easy to eat when we aren't hungry, quick to absorb and the effect is pretty much instant.

But when the blood sugar level rises, a chemical called insulin is released to normalise it again. And because the body likes to work within relatively narrow limits, any change triggers a quick reaction. In many people a sharp rise in blood sugar after a bar of chocolate means an equally sharp fall minutes later when the insulin kicks in.

This can cause moderate hypoglycaemia or low blood glucose, which explains why, after the initial good feeling you get from eating a Twix, you may be low on energy and lethargic soon afterwards. And because insulin is also related to hunger, eating that Twix may make you feel hungry again much faster than you would if you ate a chicken sandwich.

More bad news

Insulin is a storage hormone so it's harder to break down fat when you have a lot of insulin in your blood. If you eat a lot of high-sugar, refined foods that give you insulin surges, it could reduce your ability to break down fat. So not only will you be suffering from low energy levels and mood swings, you'll also be gaining weight quite rapidly.

High-glycaemic foods

All the foods on the list of simple carbohydrates in this chapter have a high sugar content and eating any of them may cause problems for people who tend to suffer from hypoglycaemia. But it's as well to be aware that there are also some Foods to Focus On which are more highly refined and contain more sugar than you might think.

FRUIT

Some fruits are naturally high in sugar, but are worth including in your diet because of their nutritional value. However, if you do have a problem with high-sugar-content foods, it's worth knowing that fruit like bananas, melon and grapes are very sweet. Also bear the following in mind:

★ Overripe fruit contains more simple sugar.
★ Fruit juices are very sweet because they are so concentrated and some even have extra sugar added to them.

VEGETABLES

We've listed potatoes under carbohydrates anyway. But, as we've already mentioned, some other vegetables such as carrots, parsnips, sweetcorn and peas contain a lot of natural sugar.

★ Cooked vegetables release their sugar content more easily than raw or undercooked ones.
★ Tinned vegetables such as baked beans, peas and even kidney beans often have added sugar, so check the label.

COMPLEX CARBOHYDRATES

Refined complex carbohydrates often have sugar added to them and the refining process means they will be absorbed more quickly into your system. Whenever you can, choose natural, wholemeal and unrefined products rather than white flour, white bread, bagels, white pasta and white rice.

HIDDEN MENACE

There are some things (usually convenience foods or pre-prepared meals) that have a surprisingly high sugar content:

★ Cooking sauces
★ Dressings and marinades
★ Dried fruit (even ones not covered in sugar)
★ Sauces and ketchup
★ Slimming, diet, 'lite' and 'lo-fat' foods
★ Snacks and bars from health food shops
★ Spreads

Compromise

Of course, you are going to use your own judgement about all this and it's often going to involve something dieters dread – a compromise. If you've been slimming for years you're probably comfortable with bingeing and starving. Swinging from one to the other may not be much fun – but it's familiar and you don't have to make so many choices. But now it's time to change. If you have to choose between two foods, neither of which is ideal, don't decide that if you can't be perfect you'll blow it for the rest of the day and go for the worst option. If it's a choice between a cheese sandwich or a plate of chips, go for the sandwich. You can't eat perfectly all the time, so make the best choice you can and enjoy it. Compromise is not a dirty word, it can be the key to success.

A NOTE ABOUT MINERALS

When you go into the health food shop or even the local chemist and see the shelves full of mineral supplements, it's tempting to think perhaps you should be taking some of those wonder tablets yourself. If you think you might have a deficiency of some kind, check with your doctor, but the chances are that if you have a varied diet and eat lots of fresh foods you will be getting all the nutrients you need.

Calcium
Dried beans
Green vegetables
Peanuts
Salmon
Sardines
Soya beans
Sunflower seeds
Walnuts
Dairy products

Magnesium
Beetroot
Egg yolk
Green leafy vegetables
Nuts
Peas
Wholegrain cereals

Sodium
Artichokes
Bacon
Carrots
Kidney
Shellfish
Vegetables

Potassium
Bananas
Citrus fruits
Green, leafy vegetables
Mint
Potatoes
Sunflower seeds
Watercress

Dieting and nutrition

Lastly and, of course, most important is the relationship between dieting and nutrition.

HOW MANY CALORIES DO YOU REALLY NEED?

★ How old are you?
★ How active are you?
★ What is your lifestyle like?
★ How tall are you?
★ How long is a piece of string?

It's hard to believe that anyone would be so simple-minded as to set hard-and-fast rules for calorie intake. But commercial diets have always worked this way and a lot of them still do. They exploit the demand for fast results and set calorie intake levels so low as to be dangerous in some cases. Of course, another word for this is undereating. And, as we explained in Chapter Two, undereating simply causes fat loss and muscle loss, which is pretty pointless because your body starts accumulating fat again as soon as your calorie levels creep up. This is because when you start using up your fat reserves too quickly, your body recognises this as an attack on its energy reserve and immediately takes defensive action so as to preserve its precious stores of fat. This is how it works:

★ Your body increases the quantity and activity of an enzyme called lipoprotein lipase – the main enzyme it uses to collect and store fat.

★ It then slows your base level metabolic rate, which reduces your fat-burning ability.

TAKE IT EASY

So if you don't want to turn your body into a battleground, take it easy. Work with your system rather than stressing it and make gentle changes to your eating habits rather than drastic cutbacks. Support your newly balanced diet with regular comfortable exercise and you'll feel a difference before you start to see it.

Take a little time and you will start to *see* some very pleasing changes in yourself as well as on your Food Profile. And it won't be just your new shape that's emerging. Your muscle tone, your skin, your hair and your energy levels will soon be reflecting the care and respect you're giving yourself now.

CHAPTER EIGHTEEN

FEEL-GOOD FITNESS

It is always advisable to check with your doctor before embarking on this or any other diet and fitness programme. Most people will benefit from undertaking exercise, but do check with your doctor if you feel that there may be some doubt as to your suitability.

THE KEY TO SUCCESS

The main reason that the British are getting fatter in spite of eating less is that we aren't taking enough exercise.[1] But in spite of the fact that we're constantly being told to be more active, most of us still aren't doing anything about it.

In 1995 the Health Education Authority reported that exercise was a key factor in managing obesity. They found too, that it greatly reduces diabetes, coronary heart disease, cancer and osteoporosis, and is even helpful to people suffering from depression. Sadly, the same report also concluded that only 36 per cent of men and 24 per cent of women were active enough to

1 UK Government National Food Survey, March 2000.

stay healthy – even though the recommended levels of exercise weren't particularly strenuous. The guidelines used were:

★ at least 30 minutes of moderate-intensity activity on at least five days a week to achieve health benefits to minimise mortality (Fat Jar Fitness).

★ at least 20 minutes of vigorous-intensity activity on three or more days a week, which maximises aerobic fitness as well as reducing mortality (Feel Good Fitness).

To make matters worse, most sedentary people didn't even know they had a problem. Fifty-six per cent of the men and 52 per cent of the women in the HEA survey actually believed they were getting plenty of exercise.[2] Findings like this show how little we know about ourselves – or perhaps how little we give our bodies the respect and attention they deserve. Our bodies were designed to move and the more we use them in the way they were intended, the better we are going to look and feel.

SLIM IS NOT ENOUGH

At Lighten Up we hardly ever say the word 'slim' without adding 'fit and healthy'. Rigid dieting or over-exercising may make you temporarily slim but it won't make you fit and healthy. Permanent slimness only happens when you work with your body and treat it well, giving it the food and exercise it needs. And a side-effect of being permanently slim is often health and fitness.

HEALTH AND FITNESS

Of course, health and fitness don't always go together, but the key to becoming slim and staying slim is to achieve both. The World Health Organisation in 1946 defined health as *'A complete state of mental, physical and social well-being not merely the absence of disease'*.

Fitness is harder to pin down, but functional fitness is usually defined as being able to carry out daily tasks without feeling

2 Health Education Authority, 1995, ISBN 0 7521 0551 5.

exhausted and recovering quickly when you do get tired. You might take a moment or two to answer these questions – don't pause to think about how you might have answered them before, just give the first answers that come to mind.

★ What does being slim mean to you now?
★ What does being healthy mean to you now?
★ What does being fit mean to you now?

SLIM, FIT AND HEALTHY

The bottom line is that slim, fit and healthy go together. It's possible to be healthy without being particularly slim or fit – but it's unusual and it's unlikely to last. If you're healthy, you're more likely to exercise and being fit certainly lowers your risk of illness. Many people believe that you can't really have one without the other two – but only you can decide whether you really want them at all.

WHERE ARE YOU STARTING FROM?

★ Do you think you are fitter and healthier now than you were when you started the Lighten Up programme?
★ How much Fat Jar activity (brisk fifteen-minute walks, bike rides etc.) are you fitting into every day?
★ Have you added some Feel Good Fitness sessions (more strenuous exercise for its own sake) into your weekly routine?
★ Are you as fit as you'd like to be yet?
★ If not, how do you know that you aren't fit enough?
★ What would you like to be able to do that you can't do now?
★ What is it that stops you from taking more exercise at the moment?
★ What could you do, starting today, to become fitter and more active?

Of course, you may already be well on the way to being fitter and healthier, but if you'd like some basic pointers to get you started, here they are.

FITNESS THAT MAKES *YOU* FEEL GOOD

First of all, we should emphasise that there is no substitute for the Fat Jar Fitness you're incorporating into your daily life. Walking and cycling when you would previously have gone by car or bus, climbing stairs instead of taking lifts and taking regular mini exercise breaks when you are sitting for long periods are all vital habits for life.

But, if you really want to lose weight and build the kind of muscle that burns fat more efficiently it's a good idea to introduce some regular Feel Good Fitness sessions into your weekly routine. In this chapter we offer some advice about what kind of exercise will get results, and explain the criteria that will help you decide what is going to work best for you.

The best kind of exercise for you

As we've explained before, Feel Good Fitness just means exercising vigorously enough to work up a sweat for half an hour to an hour three or four times a week (you can do more if you want). This chapter has a lot to say about fitness clubs and resistance training but that's only to illustrate how a successful Feel Good Fitness programme can be designed and set up. Our message is that the best kind of exercise for you is whatever you find it easiest to do on a regular basis. And there are plenty of different activities to choose from – in Week Three we listed 26 different ones. Whether it's a step class, or a dancing lesson, rowing, jogging, swimming, abseiling, cycling, athletics or any kind of sport, if it's going to work for you in the long term, choose something you can enjoy. You may like competition, you may prefer to exercise alone, at home, in the open air, or in the company of others – it's for you to decide what style suits you best.

But even if you want to go it alone in the long run, jogging in the park in the early morning, working out with baked bean tins for weights in your kitchen or moving back the furniture so that you can follow your favourite exercise video, it's a good idea to read through the rest of this chapter and get a feel for the basics before you begin.

If a fitness programme is going to help you lose weight, it will have to be individually fitted to your needs. Nobody knows you like you know yourself and, after following the Lighten Up programme for the past eight weeks, you should know yourself a lot better. Just take a moment to think through the following:

★ What are your current activity levels – including both Fat Jar Fitness and Feel Good Fitness?

★ What's your previous experience of exercising been like (assuming you have some)?

★ What are your likes and dislikes – is there anything you've tried before and hated? Or loved? Do you like team sports? Solitary walks? Swimming? Tennis? Jogging? Cycling? Rowing? Trampolining? Aerobics? Dancing?

★ How successful have you been with exercise routines in the past?

★ What's your basic attitude towards exercise? Do you think it's necessary? Or fun?

★ What are the common factors in the activities you've enjoyed before?
   ● Being alone?
   ● Competing with other people?
   ● Sharing activities – exercise with a social side?
   ● Having an audience?
   ● Being outdoors or indoors?
   ● Exercising in the morning or evening?
   ● Music? Style? Setting?
   ● .... ?
   ● .... ?

★ What are the common factors in the activities you haven't enjoyed – the ones you gave up on?
   ● .... ?
   ● .... ?

If you're just getting started on an exercise programme and it hasn't really got off the ground yet, it's always a good idea to go for something you think will be fun. If there's anything you've enjoyed doing in the past, that's a good place to start. But if there's something you've given up on in the past, don't go back there. Not yet, anyway.

If you've never had one single good exercise experience in the past, make a fresh start. Pick something you've always fancied and give it a go.

MAKE TIME FOR YOURSELF

The next thing to consider is how much time you have. Be realistic. What are you willing to give up in order to fit more exercise into your life? There are some areas where you have some leeway and some areas where you don't. If your life revolves around work, or children (or both), you may have to be creative about when, where and how you fit your exercise sessions into your life. It's definitely getting easier, though: health and fitness clubs are open early and late, and there are more of them around. Before- or after-work sessions are possible options – as are lunch-break workouts. And lots of places have crèches and children's activities where ten years ago there were none.

In fact, if you do have children, one of the most useful things you can teach them to build into their lives is the habit of fitness and enjoyment of exercise for its own sake.

RESCHEDULING YOUR LIFE

If I asked you right now whether you had any time on your hands, the chances are you'd say 'no'. In fact, you'd probably say there weren't enough hours in the day to do all the things you wanted to do.

So what are you prepared to give up in order to exercise?

★ Watching television?
★ Lying in bed?
★ Going to the pub?
★ Cleaning the house?
★ Shopping?
★ Working?
★ .... ?
★ .... ?

When you've decided how many hours a week you can set aside for exercise you are ready to make a start. And remember, you should plan in your warm-up and cool-down time (more about those later), as well as your showering, travelling and changing time. Which is why, if time is short, it's a good idea to do something that is close at hand and doesn't involve elaborate arrangements.

WORK WITH WHAT YOU'VE GOT

If your aim is to gain fitness and lose weight but you can only do a one-hour training session twice a week at the moment (and that is the absolute minimum, by the way) then just work with what you've got. However, you should realise that two hours out of one hundred and sixty-eight isn't a lot, and you will have to work hard to see any results from it. Exercising more often so that you won't have to push yourself as hard is much better. And, in fact, just a little bit of extra time can make a big difference. So before you decide that you can only budget a couple of hours, do some creative thinking and see if you couldn't free up a little bit more time – it's definitely worth it.

Finding your style

The question people always ask a fitness instructor first is, 'What's the best way to get results?'

What they really mean is 'What's the *easiest* way to get results?'

Everybody wishes there were a minimum-sweat programme that would make them as fit as Sally Gunnell in two hours a week. And, of course, we all know it's a myth – but wouldn't it be easier if there were a simple programme that anybody could follow, week in and week out, exercising by the book and getting fabulous results? Unfortunately it doesn't work like that. We may know a lot about how the body functions, but in the end, people are individuals and they all react differently to both eating and exercise.

The answer to the original question is that once you've worked out a routine that fits your lifestyle you will start to see the changes you're looking for and the feedback from that – as well as the endorphins you'll generate – will keep you going. But before you rush out and join a club, or go jogging, read through the rest of this chapter to find out what kind of programme is going to be most effective for *you*.

AEROBICS OR RESISTANCE?

Aerobic training (getting your heart rate up so that more oxygen is pumped around your body) and resistance training (toning your muscles by using weights) are the two main types of Feel Good Fitness exercise. But don't be put off by the terminology – you can do them both without any pain or humiliation and without going anywhere near a gym.

Aerobic training alone won't keep you slim so you need to do some resistance training as well. Your exercise programme should be varied and the great thing about resistance training is that it's easy to vary. Variety in exercise is important because it keeps your body guessing and surprises it out of hanging on to the status quo. Constant change and challenge is the key to success.

THE TRAINING EFFECT

When you start something new, whether it's power-walking or press-ups, it's going to be hard at first. But the more you do it, the more efficient you become, until you reach the point of easily being able to achieve your training goal every time. This usually happens between four to six weeks after starting a new exercise programme and it's called the training effect. If you want to go on getting maximum benefit from your Feel Good Fitness, then it's a good idea to do something different as soon as you start to experience that training effect. Your body regularly needs new challenges and a new stimulus to keep developing muscle and burning fat.

But don't panic. This doesn't mean that every time a training routine gets too easy you have to increase the time and intensity – if you did that you'd end up training 24 hours a day. You get round the training effect simply by varying your routine – in other words, be prepared to keep changing it. That way neither your body nor your mind will get bored.

LIVING WITH CHANGE

There's no perfect, permanent exercise routine that you can do every day for the rest of your life that will keep you slim. It might help if you think of exercise in the same way as you now think about food and include a wide variety rather than limiting your options.

Principles of training

The following formula helps you make sure you're exercising effectively. The FITT principles of training apply whether you're a top athlete or an absolute beginner. If you take each of these factors into account when you are setting up your new exercise programme, you are much more likely to be successful.

Frequency	How many times a week are you exercising?
Intensity	How hard are you exercising?
Type	Are you doing classes? Or jogging? Or playing tennis?
Time	How long is each session?
Recovery	How long do you have to recover between sessions?
Adherence	How are you going to make sure you stick with this exercise programme?

Suppose, for example, you were to go to the same aerobic class three times a week and work out for an hour at the same sort of intensity every time. Your body would adapt very quickly to that and you would reach a point where it wouldn't change. You might still be sweating away and enjoying the class, but after about three or four weeks you wouldn't be losing any more weight.

This is where the FITT principles come in handy. You can use them as the basis for a regular review of your exercise programme, changing one or other of these variables fairly regularly to make sure you stay on track and don't get into a rut. You can alternate between different types and levels of exercise, and adjust the intensity of your workouts or the length of the sessions so that your body (and your mind) don't get bored.

Aerobic training

Aerobic fitness is a measure of the body's ability to use oxygen and aerobic exercise means continuous rhythmical activity such as swimming, jogging, cycling, walking and, of course, aerobic classes. The aim is to get the cardiovascular system (heart and blood vessels) pumping blood around the body and the respiratory system taking in the oxygen that's needed to exercise intensively for long periods.

Aerobic training alone won't keep you as slim as you'd like to be but it's still a vitally important part of weight management. It's a great way to burn calories and it will speed up your metabolism as well.

SPEEDING UP YOUR METABOLISM

Your metabolism is the sum total of all the chemical reactions happening in your body at any one time and it's usually measured in terms of the number of calories used – the higher the metabolic rate the more calories you are using. During aerobic exercise the metabolic rate dramatically increases and so you use more calories. It's often called calorie *burning* because heat is a by-product of exercise, so when your workout is making you hot and sweaty that's a very good sign!

EXERCISE SIGNS

Remember the Borg Scale in Chapter Twelve? By now you should be using this simple scale quite comfortably as a way of judging how hard you're working when you exercise. However, here are some more exercise signs which will help you recognise whether you're working hard enough (and get you to slow down if you're working too hard).

★ Being able to talk but pausing for breath between sentences. If you have to breathe between words the intensity is too high; and if you can talk normally the intensity is too low.

★ Breathing very deeply through your nose. As you exercise harder you might start breathing through your mouth, but continue to breathe through your nose if you can. That's what it was designed for and you will be taking much deeper breaths that way. Mouth breathing is often shallower and you may start panting or gasping for breath, which you shouldn't need to do. However, some people really can't breathe properly through their noses and if you're one of them, don't worry about it. Just breathe in through your nose and out through your mouth.

★ Feeling you are in a rhythm and that you can go on exercising like this for a long time.

★ Sweating profusely can be an exercise sign but bear in mind that levels of sweating are quite individual. Some people sweat a lot even during low-intensity activity, while others need to work hard to build up a sweat.

★ Getting red in the face is like sweating – it depends on the individual and also on the ambient temperature at the time.

When you first start exercising it usually feels very hard, simply because it's a new challenge for your body. This is normal, but it's important to notice when you get beyond what is normal and stop.

If you start to labour, or begin to lose your rhythm, and if you suddenly start to feel it's getting much, much harder, pay attention to the warning signs: slow down and cool down.

When your workouts start to seem easier, four weeks or so into your programme and you realise you're getting the training effect, you'll know that your body has already adapted to the new demands you're putting on it. You'll find you can exercise longer and at a higher intensity and, the fitter you get, the harder you'll have to work before the exercise signs kick in. Listen to your body and, if it's telling you to do more, either work a little longer or vary the number and type of exercises you're doing. This is a good reason for starting your exercise programme in a gym where there are experts on hand to help and advise you on what to do when you reach a plateau or feel you're ready to change your routine.

HOW LONG?

The basic benchmark is a minimum of 20 minutes for any form of aerobic exercise, but as you increase your aerobic fitness you'll soon find you're able to go on longer than that. Don't worry, the fact that you will feel the training effect doesn't mean you have to keep doing longer and longer sessions – 40 minutes to an hour is enough. Just make sure you vary your activity and intensity.

Resistance training

Once you've made a start with some regular aerobic Feel Good Fitness, you might consider adding in some resistance training as well. Also known as weight training, it will help you maintain that slimmer shape, which should already be starting to emerge. Weight training doesn't need to take up much time and you don't have to join a club to do it. It's a good idea to take professional advice when you first start, but once you've got the hang of it, there is plenty of good-quality compact equipment from weights to resistance bands that you can use at home.

THE FEMALE MYTH

Resistance training is more often associated with serious athletes and body builders than with slimming – especially by women – but it's absolutely vital to long-term success.

Many women still seem to think that aerobic classes are the best way to lose body fat and they worry that using machines will turn them into the Incredible Hulk. But, if it were that simple, all the men who weight train would look like Arnold Schwarzenegger – and of course they don't. It's actually quite difficult for men to put on significant amounts of muscle. And it's even more difficult for women because the most important factor in muscle gain is the male hormone testosterone.

So now *that* myth is out of the way you can pick up your weights and start pumping.

MEN AND WOMEN

There are some very good reasons why both men and women should take up resistance training:

★ Raising self-confidence.
★ Improving posture and even correcting bad posture.
★ Making you look good.
★ Increasing bone density, which is particularly important for women nearing the menopause. Resistance training plus good nutrition helps prevent osteoporosis.
★ Strengthening the immune system.
★ Expanding the range of movement around joints.
★ Allowing you to work on specific parts of your body. Although there's no such thing as spot fat reduction you *can* work on particular muscles.
★ Increasing your resting metabolic rate so that you burn more calories even when you aren't exercising. There are two main reasons for this:
   a *Afterburn:* Muscles that have been worked in a training session require energy (calories) to build up and recover for the next session. This doesn't happen immediately and, in fact, muscle can take from 24 to 72 hours to recover completely. We aren't usually aware of this process because it doesn't require our conscious participation. The number of calories you burn after exercising will depend on the amount of effort you put into your workout. This is called the 'afterburn' of resistance exercise.
   b *Toning:* The more toned muscle you have, the higher your resting metabolic rate will be. A toned muscle is a stimulated or well-worked muscle. This isn't body-*building*, it's body *toning*.

RESISTANCE TRAINING TIPS

Here are some basic tips to get you started but if you aren't familiar with weight training or resistance machines you must get expert advice before you start, and it's better to work with a trainer until you know what you're doing. Once you've got the hang of it, you can carry on resistance training at home in your own time.

Stick to the form

Whether you're a novice or an expert, it's vital to stick to the 'form' or correct technique your instructor teaches you. If you're in the middle of lifting some weights and find you're deviating from the form, it's usually a sign that you're using too much weight and your muscles can't cope. This is dangerous and it's one of the main causes of injury. If you ever feel unsure, ask for help straight away.

★ *Repetition*: A repetition in weight training means simply lifting the weight and lowering it again – a complete up-and-down movement.
★ *Set*: You will be given a number of repetitions and a resistance weight to work with. This is called a set.
★ *Time*: It's a good idea to establish a time allowed for each repetition (or get your trainer to do it for you). This will help you to maintain your technique. As you get tired you may notice that each repetition lasts for a shorter time, which means the weight is too heavy. As a rule of thumb, try two seconds on the up phase and two seconds on the down phase, and pay particular attention to your last few repetitions.

Training effect

Look out for this – it works in exactly the same way as it does in aerobic training. After a while your body gets used to a particular weight and number of repetitions, and what seemed hard at first will start to get easier. Your muscles should feel tired at the end of each set in any type of resistance training and if this isn't happening, you aren't working them hard enough. Keep challenging your body by increasing the weights until you feel the fatigue in your muscles.

WARNING SIGNS

★ being unable to complete your set;
★ speeding up;
★ using bad form.

These are all signs that the weight is too heavy for you and that you need to reduce it.

THE FITT PRINCIPLES

Use the FITT principles to keep challenging your body. When things get easier simply adjust one of the training variables – the weights or repetitions. If you don't know which training variable to change, take your instructor's advice.

CHOOSING A CLUB

The chances are that if we've convinced you to take up resistance training, you'll want to begin by joining a club and this is what we recommend to get yourself started. That way you are much less likely to injure yourself and you'll learn the 'form' right from the beginning. If you choose a really good club with top-class instructors you will have a programme designed for you, and your heart rate as well as your progress will be regularly monitored. Then, when you're confident and you know what you're doing, you can be more flexible and do your resistance training at home.

There are plenty of clubs to choose from now and you should take the time to visit several of them and make comparisons before you decide which one to go for. Here's what you should be looking for:

Staff
★ Do they seem happy? Have a chat with them and if they don't want to chat, don't join!
★ Are there plenty of staff around? Or is it hard to find someone to answer your questions?
★ Check out their qualifications and their experience – some clubs employ much more highly skilled trainers than others.
★ Ask about the club's policy on using trainees. Of course they have to learn somewhere, but you are entitled to get your advice – especially as a beginner – from someone who is qualified and experienced.

Equipment

★ Does the equipment seem to be in good condition? Appearance is quite a good indication of whether it's up-to-date and well maintained.

★ Is the gym safe? All gyms should have a health-and-safety policy but look around and see if weights are lying about – untidiness in this environment can be a safety hazard.

★ Check up on club usage times. Busy gyms often limit the use of their aerobic equipment at peak times and you need to be sure you can have access when it suits you, not when it suits them.

The training environment

★ What is the average age of staff and members? Does it look like a place where you would feel comfortable?

★ When are the busiest times?

★ What are the opening times?

★ Do their programmes suit your interests and lifestyle?

★ What do they offer? Classes, personalised programmes, fitness checks or specialised groups? You may find that there are all sorts of interesting things on offer besides weight lifting, from tap-dancing to yoga and sometimes even social activities and an Internet café.

Your situation

★ Find someone to talk to about your personal goals, expectations and experiences, and ask what they recommend for you.

★ See if you can have a free trial (normally around a week) to see how you like it.

★ Check out the membership fees:
  ● How do you pay? Up front? In instalments?
  ● Can you freeze your membership – i.e. put your time on hold if you are ill or on holiday and unable to use the club?

If you like what you hear (including the music) give it a try. Always take up a trial visit offer if there is one because it's not until you've actually used the changing rooms and worked with the staff that you can make a final decision. Check that this particular club can really give you what you want, whether it's beginner classes or early-morning sessions. Get a feel for the place and find out at first hand whether it meets your needs.

Warming up and cooling down

Whenever you do Feel Good Fitness exercise – whether it's aerobic or resistance training – always allow time at the beginning and end of your session for warming up and cooling down.

The Warm-up prepares you physically as well as mentally for the work ahead. Start your warm-up slowly and build gradually to the work rate you're aiming for. You should walk, for example, before you break into a jog. Warm-up time varies but five minutes is recommended.

The Cool-down should round off every exercise session and will help your body get back to normal. Gradually decrease the intensity of the exercise until it becomes easy, you feel you have recovered and your breathing seems normal. Aim for a minimum of five minutes, but depending on the intensity and duration of the workout this may not be enough, so take longer if you need to.

Flexibility workouts

Flexibility work (stretching) should also be part of every exercise session. You can do these stretches just after your warm-up (the pre-stretch) and just after your cool-down (the post-stretch).

Always do your stretching when your body is warm.

Stretching is good for both your body and your mind; you don't have to go to great lengths or learn exotic ways of doing it. The safest, simplest kind of stretching is called 'static' stretching and it's taught in aerobic classes and fitness clubs – so don't guess, take a lesson and learn how to do it safely.

Fitness and fat

Have you heard that you can you burn a higher percentage of fat in low-intensity workouts? It's sometimes used as an excuse to stop doing intensive workouts – in fact, it's sometimes used as an excuse to stop doing workouts altogether and that's why I'm giving it a special mention here.

In spite of the fact that it's true on one level, this isn't a good reason to scale down your exercise programme. First of all, compare these two types of activity and take a look at what happens:

LOW-INTENSITY ACTIVITY
WALKING AT 5 CALORIES PER MINUTE

% Fat	% Non-fat (mainly Carbohydrates)	Total calories for 60 minutes
70% 210 calories	30% 90 calories	300 calories

At this intensity you are burning a lower percentage of carbohydrates and a higher percentage of fat.

MODERATE-INTENSITY ACTIVITY
RUNNING AT 10 CALORIES PER MINUTE

% Fat	% Non-fat (mainly Carbohydrates)	Total calories for 60 minutes
50% 300 calories	50% 300 calories	600 calories

At this intensity you are burning a higher percentage of carbohydrates than of fat, but overall you've burned double the calories in the same amount of time.

This obviously doesn't indicate that the best way of losing fat is to work at low intensity all the time. If you sit at a desk all day you'll be burning a higher percentage of fat over carbohydrate than you would if you were active. *But the bottom line is that you still won't be burning very much of anything!*

Of course, high-intensity exercise isn't the only sort that's useful, which is why we introduced you to regular, everyday Fat Jar exercise first. Fat Jar Fitness is a habit for life, but, to become slimmer and stay that way, you want to be doing two to four Feel Good Fitness sessions every week as well.

Decision time

If you haven't already put some Feel Good Fitness into your life, you should be convinced by now. And you've got all the information you need. You know about the FITT principles of training, you know that you need a mixture of both aerobic and resistance exercise, and you know that it's a good idea to vary your programme regularly so as to stimulate the process of change.

ADHERENCE

Do you remember the last of the FITT principles – adherence? In a way, it's the most important of all. You may not have the most perfect exercise routine in the world, but if you do it regularly it will be a thousand times more valuable to you than any of the state-of-the-art ones I designed for my clients in the past but which they didn't stick to.

Do you think you can carry out and maintain these lifestyle changes by yourself? Will you need some help and support? And if you will, how are you going to get them?

GIVE YOURSELF THE SUPPORT YOU NEED

Here are a few questions that good personal trainers often ask new clients:

★ Do you like starting new things?
★ Do you always finish what you start?
★ Do you lose interest in new projects?
★ Are you focused?
★ Do you need support when you set out to achieve something?
★ If you do, who is going to support you?

- ★ Is anybody likely to try to sabotage your attempts at regular exercise?
- ★ How are you going to stop them?

This won't tell you anything you don't know, but it might just inspire you to do something about it. For example, if you know that you find it easy to start something but hard to keep going, or that you need support, build those things into your plan at the beginning. It's much better to begin with all your support structures in place than to find out after a couple of weeks that you can't get out of bed to run in the mornings because your partner keeps turning off the alarm clock, or that you can't get to the gym after work because your colleagues expect you to go with them to the pub.

Remember, there will be people in your life who will make it difficult for you. However much they love you and want you to succeed, they will still feel threatened when you put on your new running shoes and head for the park while they're still sitting at the kitchen table with a cup of tea.

Finish building the house before you move in. Solve any problems you anticipate facing well in advance. Arrange for someone to jog with you – or make a commitment to run with somebody's dog. Partner up with someone who's really motivated or who is already doing whatever it is you want to start. Think creatively about how you can make your new exercise programme crash-proof so it becomes as basic a part of your routine as brushing your teeth – something you wouldn't even consider not doing.

A relationship with life

Regular Feel Good Fitness exercise means a lot of things to a lot of people. But I've never met anyone who exercised regularly and didn't enjoy it. It's a relationship with life and a relationship *for* life. Think of it, like eating, as something you are going to do for ever. It's time spent with yourself and for yourself, an investment in your own future. For some people it's the only time they get alone to think through their day. For others it's the focus of their social life. Whatever it is for you, always look for the pleasure you're going to get out of it because it's the pleasure that will keep you going.

Of course, you won't get instant results, especially if you've got a lifetime of lethargy and self-neglect to overcome. Give yourself as much time as you need and you will see a difference – and feel it, too. There will be days when you'd rather not bother and there may be people who'll make you feel awkward or uncomfortable But in the end the only person who matters and the only person you're doing it for is you. So, make a start. And keep going.

CHAPTER NINETEEN

FEEL-GOOD FOOD

Many people with weight problems see food as a necessary evil; in fact, for some people the evil outweighs the necessity and they lose all sense of the pleasure of eating. But if you really take time to enjoy your meals and to prepare fresh food lovingly – for yourself and for others – you'll find it much harder to overeat. We hope you'll try some of the Lighten Up recipes and that you'll rediscover the joy of cooking and preparing food, and the joy of eating it as well.

THE DYNAMIC BALANCE

Forget grazing, picking, nibbling and snacking while you work. When you want to eat, think first about what you're going to have and then take time to enjoy it.

Planning your meals

Not everybody feels like planning their meals for a week – life's not like that any more. What you'll be eating tends to depend on what you'll be doing and who you'll be eating with, and you may not know that for more than a few hours in advance.

But it's a good idea to plan your day – even as you go along – so that you're sure you are getting a good balance. The Food Profile will help you with this, of course. You should be able to see at a glance whether you're mostly on target in Food to Focus On or whether everything is piling up in the takeaway segment on the Foods to Limit circle.

★ Always include your minimum of five portions of fruit or vegetables.
★ Build your meals around good (whole and unprocessed) complex carbohydrate. Try to vary this, so that you don't end up with toast for breakfast, a sandwich for lunch and pizza for dinner. That would (probably) be wheat, wheat and wheat, which isn't varied enough.
★ If you know that you're having a sandwich for lunch, plan to have fruit, cereal or yoghurt for breakfast and if you think you might be eating out in the evening, make sure you get your fruit in during the day (most restaurants don't serve much fresh fruit).

You may not be able to plan a perfect personal menu for a whole week, but with a little forward thinking you can balance what you eat day by day.

THE LIGHTEN UP STORE CUPBOARD

Back in Week Seven we suggested that you might get into the habit of shopping with intent (and a list) so that your store cupboard always has the basics for making great meals and snacks without resorting to fast food or takeaways. There's no need to get stuck with pot noodles or a bag of chips if you've done your planning in advance.

We hope that you'll be shopping more often for fresh foods, but there are some things you should always have in the larder:

★ A good range of dried herbs and spices: don't keep them too long and don't expose them to light and heat – a rack in the window or by the cooker is a really bad idea. If you can grow your own herbs that's great, but if you live in a big city you might think twice about the pollution that's going to settle all over them.

★ Cooking oil (olive oil, sunflower, safflower, sesame and borage).
★ Cereals (unsweetened basics as far as possible).
★ Dried or long-life skimmed or semi-skimmed milk or non-dairy substitute.
★ Nuts and seeds (almonds, brazils, hazelnuts, pumpkin seeds, sesame seeds, sunflower seeds, walnuts)
★ Dried fruit
★ Dried beans and lentils
★ Fresh garlic and ginger (these add flavour to lots of things and keep for quite a while in the fridge)
★ Frozen vegetables and unsweetened fruit (better than none at all)
★ Frozen meat (keep it simple, not covered in sauces or pre-prepared)
★ Pasta
★ Rice and other grains
★ Tins of tomatoes and different kinds of tinned beans
★ Tinned fish (tuna and sardines)

Always buy the best quality you can get and, wherever possible, choose wholemeal and unrefined foods.

Look at the label

Get used to reading the labels on foods you might take for granted. Look for:

★ Fat content
★ Sugar content (anything that ends in -ose)
★ Proportion of sugar to carbohydrate (i.e. simple carbo-hydrate to complex carbohydrate)
★ Additives (usually colourings, flavourings and preservatives beginning with E and followed by a number)

You'll soon find you are developing a kind of personal radar that alerts you to nasties and you will start naturally selecting the simpler, more basic foods and adding your own fresh, sugar-free flavourings.

Store cupboard food doesn't have to be over-processed, over-packaged and pre-prepared, with added fat, sugar, colouring, flavouring and preservatives. Choose basic dried foods and frozen foods, and always check tinned-food labels for added salt, sugar and oil.

Dynamic leftovers

Leftovers are a great idea. For a start, if it's left over it means you probably resisted the temptation to overeat – so, congratulations!

There are two things you can do with leftovers:

1 Freeze them (because then they keep longer and you can't just pick them out of the freezer and eat them on impulse without defrosting them first).

2 Rename them *'personally pre-prepared meals'* and think how much time and effort you'll save when you have new potatoes, tomato sauces, roast vegetables and soup all ready to use in the fridge.

THE LIGHTEN UP KITCHEN

Cooking style

★ Eat some of your vegetables raw or lightly cooked.
★ Boil, steam or grill your food rather than frying it.
★ Limit the use of oil, choose good-quality oils like olive oil and don't overheat them. When even good-quality oils are overheated they break down into forms that aren't so good for you. Of course, you need to heat them up to cook in them, but when you're frying or grilling food with oil, do it quickly and lightly. Avoid oil-filled deep-fat fryers that cook at high temperatures and re-use oil.

★ Use herbs and spices to enhance the flavour of food rather than salt and sugar (the two great British standbys). We are gradually becoming more adventurous with exotic flavours in our cooking but we could learn a lot from Chinese and Indian cuisine. It's a pity that takeaways have given curries and stir-fries such a bad name because these foods can be just as delicious and much healthier when they are prepared at home using less fat and more fresh vegetables. So if you haven't experimented before, buy yourself some oriental cookery books and get some fresh ideas for using rice rather than chips.

Kitchens are more health-food-friendly places than they've ever been before. You can store fresh food for longer and there are all kinds of gadgets and cooking aids that will help you prepare it quickly and easily without overcooking it or adding too much fat.

Useful gadgets

★ A hand-held bar or stick blender to whizz soups in the pan, purée fruits, shakes and smoothies in the glass or jug. It also makes it easy to put together your own low-fat dressings, dips and marinades with healthy ingredients and no additives.
★ A centrifugal juicer for making fruit and vegetable juices. Some people prefer their fruit and veggies intact, but a lot of people find juicing (or making smoothies) is the best way to make sure they get their five portions of fruit or vegetables every day.
★ Pump-action atomiser sprays (from kitchen shops and chemists). Fill one with oil and one with water so that you can lightly spray what you're cooking to help it brown or stay moist. Salads can be 'glazed' with a quick spray of olive oil and so can sweetcorn. These sprays deliver only a fraction of the usual drizzle from a bottle.
★ A good, heavy, non-stick frying pan is essential for dry frying and sautéing without fat.
★ A fine cheese plane, mandolin or slicer produces thinner slices than you can cut with a knife. They are great for making

sandwiches or for producing slivers of parmesan. You can also cut some very attractive-looking vegetables with them for salads.

★ A balloon or flat whisk made of plastic instead of metal so that you can use it with non-stick pans. These are fantastic for making low-fat 'instant' sauces.

★ Plastic food storage boxes for leftovers and lunches.

★ Your own cook book – either in a notebook or a card index – is much more useful and practical than stacks and stacks of recipe books you'll never use more than once. Also, when you accidentally make something that turns out well, you can write down what you did so that you can do it again.

RECIPES

The recipes in this book are all light and easy. Even the dinner party menus give you more time with your guests than in the kitchen.

They are designed to be a user-friendly introduction to enjoying food again because we know that some of you will have lost the knack of that. They are also a safety net for you in difficult times because this is the kind of food you can eat when you're alone, when you're in a hurry, or when you might otherwise be tempted to go out and get something that won't do you any good. It's the kind of food that's always available and easy to prepare, so that you don't get into that desperate 'what shall I eat – there's nothing but chocolate mousse and pizza' situation.

A lot of the recipes assume that you will have a well-stocked store cupboard. So before you start, take another look at the store cupboard suggestions, write out your own list and stock up on the basics.

All day breakfasts

Be open-minded about what foods you eat at particular mealtimes.

Eggs and bacon, for example, aren't the only way to break your overnight fast. Millions of Chinese, Vietnamese and

Indonesian people start the day on a dish of rice or noodles with aromatic flavourings. It may seem a bit exotic, but it's a lot healthier than fried bread and black pudding. So many of our breakfast eating habits have survived unchallenged simply because first thing in the morning doesn't feel like the best time to be adventurous. So we rely on what we're used to – encouraged by the big-budget advertising of the international food companies who want to sell us more extra-sugary, highly processed cereals.

Why not rethink the way you start the day and have a bowl of fresh, colourful fruit, maybe with some unsweetened cereal, topped by totally natural low-fat yoghurt? This works for lunch as well if you add an apple, banana, peach, nectarine or grapes to some muesli.

ALMOST INSTANT BREAKFASTS

★ If you prefer toast, try as many different kinds of unrefined, unprocessed bread as you can find – there's a huge variety now, including wholemeal wheat, rye and mixed grain. Or you might like to try rice cakes or crackers.

★ Omelettes are great at any time of day and you can make tortilla or frittata the basis of a packed lunch. Go easy on the egg yolks, though, they're very high in cholesterol (you can make an omelette just with white of egg).

★ Home-made muffins are great for a quick breakfast or even to take to work for break times. If you bake your own you can be sure you use the best ingredients and cut back on the sugar. Make up a batch at the weekend and freeze, ready to use one at a time.

★ Sesame Ryvita topped with cottage cheese and fresh fruit like strawberries or nectarine makes a Californian-style breakfast.

★ Sliced banana on granary toast sprinkled with cinnamon.

★ Toasted leftover baguette, rubbed with a little garlic and topped with diced tomato, salt and pepper is a breakfast favourite in many Mediterranean countries.

★ Grilled kippers with granary toast.

★ Porridge cooked with milk or soya milk and topped with chopped dates and sliced pear.

FRENCH TOAST OR 'EGGY BREAD'

A favourite from childhood, this is one dish that still deserves its place in an adult diet. It's usually served sweet but you could add some savoury flavours instead.

Makes 1 portion
Cooking time: 2–3 minutes

1 egg
2 tbsp milk
¼–½ tsp curry powder
Salt and pepper
2 slices wholemeal bread
1 tbsp chutney

In a large flat bowl beat together the first four ingredients, dip in each bread slice to soak up all the mixture.

Heat a non-stick frying pan and cook one slice at a time over medium heat until lightly browned and just firm to the touch. Spread the chutney over one slice and sandwich the two slices together.

Variations: Instead of curry powder use a little cumin or paprika. Sandwich with a little peanut butter, Marmite, diced tomato or tomato ketchup.

HOME-MADE MUESLI

Find a whole-food store that sells loose cereals and grains, and buy a variety of different ones in small amounts to try. Don't stock up with large quantities unless you really use a lot – they will be fresher if you buy them regularly.

Starting with a base of rolled oats, experiment until you find your own personalised mix. You can add lots of other grains: puffed brown rice, oatbran and wheatbran – whatever you fancy. Then add a few raisins and a few chopped nuts.

Next, soak a portion of this mixture overnight in water and, in the morning, add a few tablespoons of milk, soya milk, fruit juice or yoghurt and a chopped or grated apple.

If you've never soaked the muesli base before in the traditional way you'll find it a revelation, soaking breaks down some of the hard-to-digest starches, which makes them not only taste sweeter but also easier to absorb.

HOME-MADE GRANOLA

Like the muesli, this can be made with a huge variety of ingredients, but try this simple mixture first, then make your own additions.

350g/12oz rolled oats (porridge oats)
75g/2¾oz desiccated coconut and/or the same
amount of chopped nuts
50g/1¾oz sunflower and sesame seeds
85g/3oz each of raisins and chopped dates
3 tbsp clear honey
3 tbsp sunflower oil

Mix the first five ingredients together in a bowl.

In a small pan warm the honey with the sunflower oil, drizzle over the ingredients in the bowl and toss well to coat evenly.

Grease a baking sheet or roasting tin (or line with baking parchment).

Tip the mixture out on to the baking sheet and spread it evenly.

Bake at 180C/350F/Gas Mark 4 for about 20 minutes, stirring halfway through, until golden brown and crispy.

When cool, store in an airtight container.

BREAKFAST IN A GLASS – FRUIT SMOOTHIE

Smoothies are great for those occasions when you haven't got the time or inclination to sit down and eat a meal. You can make them with any fruit you happen to have around, so experiment until you find your favourites.

This can be a few tablespoons of live yoghurt, milk, soya milk, rice milk, *or* if you prefer, use fresh fruit juice such as apple, mango, pineapple, orange or cranberry. Pour this into the liquidiser.

Fruit

One banana plus whatever fruit is in season. It could be strawberry, raspberry, peach, nectarine, kiwi, pear, pineapple, papaya, mango, or whatever you fancy. Add this to the smoothie base in the liquidiser.

Flavouring (optional)

One tablespoon of any of these: dried skimmed milk powder, coconut milk powder, desiccated coconut, ground almonds, wheatgerm or flaxseed oil, or one teaspoon of honey. If you want to include any of these, simply add them to the mixture so far, whiz together until it's smooth, pour into a large glass and enjoy.

Soups and meals in a bowl

If you can boil a potato you can make soup, even if you've never tried before. Now that there are good-quality fresh soups sold in cartons it's easy to enjoy soup more often but they are expensive to buy. You can make your own in large batches and freeze some in individual portions ready for when you need to eat in a hurry.

For the past few years various soups have been associated with diet programmes, the Cabbage Soup diet being the most famous. The Cabbage Soup diet (or Yummy Yum diet, as it's also known) still attracts a big following by promising ten pounds of weight loss in a week. As only two pounds of that could possibly be fat there doesn't seem to be much point in it and it certainly doesn't sound like fun.

But don't let that put you off soup, because soup is great – and there's even some evidence that it really can help you lose weight.

In a recent study[1] normal-weight women were given a lunch of either chicken and rice casserole, chicken and rice casserole

1 Elizabeth Bell, Pennsylvania State University, USA, 1999.

plus a glass of water, or chicken and rice soup. The soup contained the same ingredients as the casserole but the women who ate the soup felt much fuller on fewer calories. Drinking water with the casserole made no difference. Interestingly, the ones who ate the soup didn't go on to make up the calorie deficit later in the day.

Elizabeth Bell, one of the researchers, said, 'A lot of the explanation is psychological. The women were presented with a huge bowl of food and it felt like a lot. If it could trick normal-weight women who successfully regulate their food intake, then it could be even more successful with overweight women whose food regulation is less good.'

That seems to show that the best way to lose weight is to eat normally but, where you can, substitute vegetables and watery things for fat and high-energy, dense food. But it doesn't have to be cabbage soup – in fact, from the point of view of your Food Profile, the more variety you can introduce into your soup the better.

BASIC SOUP PROPORTIONS

Be adventurous and make up your own soups with your favourite ingredients and seasonings. See what you have in the fridge or store cupboard, use leftovers and take the opportunity to buy fresh foods that are cheap and in season.

Serves 4–6
Cooking time: 15–30 minutes

500g–1kg/1lb2oz–2lb4oz solids: vegetables, canned tomatoes,
sweetcorn, beans, potatoes, rice, onions, garlic, pasta etc.
1–1.5 lt/1¾ – 2¾pt meat or vegetable stock
Seasonings, spices and flavourings

Simply sauté the chopped onion, garlic and any other hard vegetables in a tablespoon of oil to soften and turn them a light golden brown, which brings out their sweetness and flavour. Using a non-stick pan and covering it while you sauté the vegetables so that they sweat as well as fry will mean using less oil. (You can speed things up by leaving out this stage and simply cooking all the ingredients together but it won't taste quite as good.)

Next add any softer vegetables (like tomatoes) and beans, rice, pasta etc., plus the stock or water and simmer until everything is tender.

Taste and adjust the seasonings.

Decide whether you want to eat it rough and chunky, blended with a hand-held blender bar until roughly chopped with a bit of texture, or completely liquidised until it's velvety smooth.

SOUP SUGGESTIONS

★ Sweet potato, onion, garlic and a can of creamed sweetcorn with fresh coriander, lime juice and paprika or chilli.

★ Leek, potato and onion with chicken stock and low-fat crème fraiche or quark. This can be left chunky or whizzed until smooth and velvety.

★ Canned ratatouille and a drained can of cannellini beans cooked with vegetable stock, garlic salt and sweet paprika pepper, a real store cupboard standby that takes less than five minutes to make.

★ Red pepper, canned or fresh tomato and carrot with garlic and paprika.

★ Squash or pumpkin chowder with onion, potato, ginger and lime.

★ Pasta, potato and pesto soup, another rustic one which cooks in the time it takes to have a shower!

★ Carrot and coriander with onion, parsnip and lentils or a can of cannellini beans, very filling.

JAPANESE NOODLE SOUP

The quality of the stock you use really determines the finished flavour of any dish, especially in these clear soups that are more of a meal in a bowl.

Noodle bars are very fashionable places to eat but it's quite easy to cook in the same style at home. Simply cook Japanese ramen or soba noodles in good-quality stock and add your own choice of flavourings at the end of the cooking process. Some suggestions might be shredded chicken or fish, spinach leaves, pak choy, sliced mushrooms, bean sprouts, sliced leeks, celery or carrot, chopped fresh chilli, ginger and coriander leaves.

ITALIAN MAMA'S MINESTRONE

Wherever you go in Italy you will find different versions of wonderfully fragrant, thick, sustaining meal-in-a-bowl soups. A modern summer version could be made with tomato, courgette, peppers and fennel, spiked with a little chilli and the juice and rind of a lime.

Serves: 4–6
Cooking time: 20–25 minutes

750g /1lb10oz vegetables, including your own choice
of what is seasonally available, e.g. onion, garlic, carrot,
parsnip, potato, leek, celeriac, celery, cabbage,
broccoli, peppers, courgette, fennel
1.5lt/2¾pt vegetable stock
400g/14oz-can chopped tomatoes
75g/ 2¾oz small pasta shapes for soup or
quick-cook macaroni
Seasoning

Garnish:
chopped fresh herbs and a little freshly grated
parmesan cheese

Chop the vegetables into small dice or rough and chunky pieces, whichever you prefer, and place in a large pan.

Add the stock, canned tomatoes and pasta, bring to the boil and simmer for 15–20 minutes, or until the vegetables and pasta are tender and the soup is thick.

Taste and adjust the seasoning, and serve garnished with herbs and a sprinkling of parmesan.

TOMATO AND BASIL SOUP

Serves 2
Cooking time: 25 minutes

1 tsp olive oil
200g/7oz chopped plum tomatoes
1 tsp garlic purée
1 tsp tomato purée
300ml vegetable or beef stock
Salt and pepper
1 good handful of fresh basil, chopped

Heat the olive oil in a large saucepan. Then add the tomatoes, the garlic purée and the tomato purée. Lower the heat and leave to simmer gently for about 10 minutes.

Stir in the stock and leave to simmer for a further 10 minutes. Season to taste.

Stir in three-quarters of the basil and either pour into a food processor or liquidiser, or use a hand blender to turn this into a smooth soup (alternatively you can just leave it chunky).

Serve garnished with the rest of the basil.

SPANISH SOPA DI PICADILLO

Picadillo usually refers to a salad of diced vegetables, but here the vegetables are used to make a rich, satisfying broth or soup, with rice and Spanish Serrano ham, bacon or gammon. Vegetarians can leave out the meat and it will still taste good.

Serves 4
Cooking time: 20–25 minutes

1–2 tbsp olive oil
1 medium onion, carrot and potato, diced
100g/3½oz paella or risotto rice
1lt/1¾ pt additive-free chicken or vegetable stock
50g/1¾oz Serrano ham, chopped
Juice and rind of ½ lemon
Salt and sweet red paprika pepper
1–2 tbsp chopped fresh mint

Heat the oil in a large pan and add the vegetables; sauté for a few minutes, stirring, before adding the rice.

Add the stock, bring to the boil, reduce the heat, cover and simmer for 15–20 minutes until the rice is just tender.

Add the chopped Serrano ham, lemon juice, seasoning and mint, and serve.

Variations: Instead of Serrano ham you can use the equally low-fat Italian prosciutto or Parma ham, or grilled lean bacon, bacon lardons or gammon.

This dish can be made even more quickly using leftover rice or even canned white or brown long-grain rice, in which case you would need to reduce the amount of stock you use.

Light meals

MACARONI AND BROCCOLI CHEESE

A new take on an old favourite adds vegetables like cauliflower, broccoli or leeks to the macaroni to make it a cross between cauliflower cheese and macaroni cheese, made with an easy, low-fat 'instant' sauce.

Serves 4
Cooking time: 10–20 minutes

200g/7oz macaroni (you can use quick-cook
if you're in a hurry)
450g/1lb broccoli, cauliflower, leek etc.
600ml/1pt semi-skimmed milk, or
half milk half vegetable stock
50g/1¾oz plain flour
75g/2¾oz mature strong cheddar
1 tsp smooth Dijon mustard
Salt and pepper

Cook the pasta in a large pan of boiling salted water, until just tender or 'al dente'.

If possible cook the broccoli in a steamer over the pasta, or simmer in a little water until just tender. Drain and keep hot.

Put the milk and flour into a non-stick pan and heat slowly, whisking continuously with a plastic or nylon whisk, until the sauce thickens, then add the cheese, mustard and seasonings.

Add the broccoli and sauce to the cooked drained pasta and mix it together gently.

Variation: If you're not aiming to have a particularly low-fat meal, add a tablespoon of vegetable oil to the milk and flour for the sauce.

SALMON WITH CREAMY WATERCRESS SAUCE

Serves 4
Cooking time: 6–8 minutes

4 salmon fillets
1 tbsp olive oil
1 bunch spring onions, finely sliced
1 bunch or bag watercress, washed
and roughly chopped
1 tbsp lemon juice
4 tbsp low fat soft cheese

Simply grill or griddle the salmon for a few minutes each side, until just firm and lightly golden brown.

Meanwhile, in a small pan heat the olive oil and sauté the spring onions until softened, then add the watercress and cook until just wilted. Add any juices from the cooked salmon and the lemon juice, and cook for a further 30 seconds.

Add the soft cheese and, using a hand-held bar blender, purée the sauce until smooth, season and taste.

Serve the salmon with a little sauce on the side.

CHICKEN AND RED PEPPER KEBABS
WITH SALAD AND PITTA BREAD

Serves 2
Cooking time: 30 minutes

2 skinless chicken breast fillets, cut into large cubes
1 onion, cut into 8 large pieces
1 red pepper, cut into large dice
Pitta bread and green salad

Marinade:
1 tsp wholegrain mustard
½ tbsp olive oil
½ tbsp white wine vinegar
25g/1oz fresh coriander, chopped
Dash of Tabasco sauce (optional)

If you are using wooden kebab skewers, first soak them in water for about 10 minutes to stop them from burning when they are under the grill.

Mix together the marinade ingredients.

Thread the chicken, onion and red pepper chunks alternately on to the skewers.

Place the kebabs on a large plate and pour over the marinade. Roll the kebabs in the marinade using your hands to make sure that all the chicken and vegetables are well coated.

Cover the kebabs and place them in the fridge for 30–60 minutes.

Preheat the grill to high and cook the kebabs for 15–20 minutes, turning three times.

When the kebabs appear to be well cooked on all sides, check that the chicken is cooked through properly. You can do this by slicing open one of the pieces – it should be white all the way through.

Serve with pitta bread and a green salad.

The next three recipes all use avocados – a fruit which often frightens slimmers who think it's high in calories. In fact, the calorie content is more than justified by its food value, the fat it contains is monounsaturated, it's full of protein, vitamins A, E and B, and potassium, and it's nutritious enough to form the main part of a meal.

PRAWN AND AVOCADO SALAD WITH CORIANDER DRESSING

Serves 2

115g/4oz mixed salad leaves
1 avocado – peeled and sliced
200g/7oz prawns
1 red pepper – grilled, skinned and sliced*
2 tbsp extra virgin olive oil
1 tbsp Dijon mustard
2 tbsp lemon juice
4 tbsp crème fraiche or low-fat yoghurt
2 handfuls fresh coriander – finely chopped
Salt and freshly milled black pepper

Arrange the salad leaves on individual plates with the avocado, prawns and strips of red pepper on top, then whisk the rest of the ingredients together to make the dressing. Drizzle 2 tablespoons of the creamy dressing over each salad and pass the extra dressing round if you want.

Serve with fresh wholemeal bread and sliced tomatoes with chopped chives.

* You can buy peppers in jars, but they tend to be very oily so it's better to skin your own. Skewer the pepper with a fork at one end and hold it in the flame of a gas burner or under an electric grill. The skin will bubble and, when it's black all over, let it cool for a couple of minutes. The skin should peel away pretty easily and then you can slice it up.

BACON AND AVOCADO SALAD WITH A
WARM TOMATO AND BASIL VINAIGRETTE

Serves 2

4 rashers bacon (smoked or unsmoked,
chopped into smallish pieces)
115g/4oz mixed salad leaves or rocket
1 avocado, peeled and sliced
Small handful black olives
1 tbsp olive oil
1 shallot or ¼ onion – finely chopped
2 handfuls fresh basil – roughly chopped
5 tbsp balsamic vinegar
Pinch of sugar
Freshly milled black pepper

Fry the bacon in a pan over moderate heat (if you have a non-stick pan there's no need for any extra oil). When it's crispy, drain the fat on some kitchen roll.

Arrange the salad leaves, avocado, olives and bacon on individual plates.

Make the dressing by heating the olive oil in a saucepan until it just starts to bubble, then add the shallot or onion and the basil. Let it bubble for a minute and add the balsamic vinegar and sugar. (Don't leave it on for long – olive oil should be heated to the minimum). Season with black pepper.

Drizzle 2 tablespoons over each salad and pass the rest round.

Serve with fresh wholemeal bread.

TONNO E FAGIOLI

This is a variation on an Italian classic. It makes a great supper, or you can make it the night before and put it into a plastic box for lunch the next day. It's packed full of energy and should keep you going all day.

Serves 2

400g/14oz tin cannellini beans, drained
400g/14oz tin borlotti beans, drained
½ red onion finely sliced
200g/7oz tin tuna in brine, drained
1 avocado – peeled and chopped into largish chunks
5 tbsp extra virgin olive oil
2 tbsp red-wine vinegar
2 tsp dried oregano
Salt and pepper

Mix all the ingredients together and that's it. You can add chopped red peppers, cooked green beans, sweetcorn or olives, and you can increase the quantity of tuna. But the beans and dressing make a great base. If you're concerned about the avocado going brown, toss it in lemon juice or add it just before you're ready to eat.

TUNA AND BEAN SALAD

Here's an even speedier, though rather more humble, version of 'Tonno e Fagioli'. Use flaked fresh tuna or a can of tuna in brine or spring water instead of oil.

To this add a drained can of flageolet or cannellini beans and a small red onion thinly sliced. Serve on a bed of mixed salad leaves with a low-fat dressing, plenty of freshly chopped parsley and crusty bread.

CURRIED SMOKED HADDOCK
AND BASMATI RICE

This is a great dish all the family can enjoy. Curry freaks can increase the heat at will, or to make a more economical dish reduce the amount of fish used and add a drained can of butter beans or chickpeas.

Serves : 4
Cooking time: 15–20 minutes

450g/1lb uncoloured smoked haddock, skinned
1 tbsp oil
1 onion, chopped
2 sticks celery, chopped
1 tbsp mild curry powder
½ tsp turmeric
1 tbsp sweet chilli sauce or few shakes Tabasco
280g/10oz basmati rice
140g/5oz frozen petits pois
Pepper
4 tbsp chopped fresh parsley or coriander
1 lemon

Cut the fish into 3–4 pieces to fit into a large saucepan more easily in one layer, then pour over enough boiling water just to cover. Bring to the boil, reduce the heat and simmer for 4 minutes. Drain off and retain the liquid, cover the fish and keep hot.

Clean the pan and add the oil; allow to heat before adding the onion and celery. Cook together for a few minutes to soften and just begin to brown. Add the curry powder and turmeric, and continue to cook, stirring for a minute before adding the chilli sauce and rice. Stir together for another minute.

Make the retained fish stock up to 600ml/1pt with water and add to the pan, bring to the boil then reduce the heat and simmer for about 10 minutes until the stock is almost all absorbed and the rice is tender. Add the petit pois 2–3 minutes before the end of cooking time.

Add more stock or water during cooking, as necessary, and the pepper.

Serve sprinkled with herbs and wedges of lemon, with Indian breads and a green salad.

TURKEY MINCE BOLOGNESE

Turkey meat, minced without any skin, is one of the leanest meats you can choose, as well as being an excellent source of protein. Why not make double the amount and freeze some in individual portions for future use.

Serves 4–6
Cooking time: 20–25 minutes

1 tbsp oil
1 large onion, chopped
3–4 cloves garlic, sliced or chopped
450g/1lb minced turkey
2 large carrots, peeled and grated
600ml/1pt tomato passata or chopped tomatoes
2 tbsp tomato purée
1 tsp mixed herbs
300ml/½pt stock
Salt and pepper

In a large saucepan heat the oil over a medium heat and sauté the onion and garlic. Stir while they're softening and just beginning to brown. Add the minced turkey and over a high heat stir quickly to brown lightly. Add the carrots, tomato passata, purée, herbs, stock and a little seasoning.

Reduce the heat and simmer for about 20 minutes until the sauce is rich and thick, adding a little more stock or water if necessary. Taste and adjust seasoning.

Use as a stuffing for vegetables like peppers, tomatoes, marrow or courgettes, or serve with pasta, polenta or garlic mashed potatoes.

VEGETABLE FRITTATA

Frittatas are extremely versatile. Try with different vegetables and even pasta. All are excellent served hot or cold, making an interesting packed lunch or picnic ingredient.

Serves 4
Cooking Time: 15–20 minutes

2 tbsp oil
2 fat cloves garlic, chopped
1 onion, thinly sliced
1 large or 2 small courgettes, sliced

2 small red and/or yellow peppers, deseeded and chopped
1 small can sweetcorn, drained
6 medium eggs
3 tbsp chopped fresh herbs
Salt and pepper

Heat the oil in a large non-stick frying pan, then add the garlic, onion, courgette and peppers; stir-fry until the vegetables are softened and beginning to brown. This will take at least 5 minutes.

Add the sweetcorn and stir in.

Beat the eggs in a bowl with the herbs and seasoning, pour over the vegetables in the pan and reduce the heat to low.

Cook slowly for about 10 minutes until almost all the egg is set and the base is golden brown. Meanwhile preheat the grill. Place the pan under the grill to finish cooking the top of the frittata. (Take care to cover the pan handle if necessary.)

Serve wedges of the frittata with crusty bread. It is great eaten either hot or cold.

ROASTED HERB-CRUSTED COD

Serves 4
Cooking time: 15 minutes

4 chunky cod fillets
2 tbsp olive oil
1 lime, juice and finely grated rind
3 tbsp parsley, chopped
3 tbsp chives, finely chopped
1 tsp smooth French mustard
Salt and pepper
125g/4½oz fresh breadcrumbs

Preheat the oven to 220C/425F/Gas Mark 7. Lightly grease an ovenproof dish big enough to take the fish with a little space around each piece. Arrange the fish in the dish.

To make the herb crust, place all the remaining ingredients in a bowl and mix thoroughly. Divide over each piece of fish, pressing on lightly.

Bake in the oven, uncovered for about 15 minutes or until the fish is firm to the touch and cooked through.

Variations: Different flavours can be added to the crust: try grated fresh ginger and spring onion instead of chives, or 1 tablespoon finely grated parmesan cheese.

CHICKEN AND BROCCOLI WITH RICE

Serves 4
Cooking time: 20 minutes

225g/8oz broccoli florets
1 tbsp vegetable oil
1 onion, chopped
2 courgettes, sliced
125g/4½oz button mushrooms, sliced
2 tbsp plain flour
150ml/¼pt semi-skimmed milk
150ml/¼pt chicken or vegetable stock
350g/12oz cooked leftover chicken

Steam the broccoli florets over a pan of boiling water until tender.

Heat the oil in a large saucepan and add the onion, cook for 2–3 minutes to soften. Add the courgettes and mushrooms, and sauté together, stirring frequently over a medium heat for 5–6 minutes until the vegetables are almost tender.

Sprinkle over the flour and stir in, then add the milk and stock. Bring to the boil and stir gently until the mixture has thickened.

Add the broccoli and chicken and simmer gently for 4–5 minutes; taste and season as necessary. Serve with rice.

VERY QUICK AND EASY MEALS

★ Polenta with Gorgonzola: sounds absolutely decadent, but it doesn't have to be forbidden. Make quick-cook polenta (see page 413) with additive-free vegetable stock, then top it with a slice of cheese (use about 25g/1oz per person), melt under the grill and serve with lots of wilted spinach with Garlic Sauce (see below).

★ Spicy almond couscous (cooked according to the packet instructions), with vegetables and Middle Eastern flavours, fruit and nuts.

★ Vegetable stir-fry with rice noodles, prawns, chicken or tofu.

★ Tuna and sweetcorn potato cakes.

Dips, dressings and salads

These can be amazingly sensual when you combine the right colours, flavours and smells. Salads and crudités served with lovely dips and dressings are wonderful in summer, but you can have them in winter too. Many dips can be turned into dressings by simply adding enough milk or water to give a pouring or spooning consistency.

GARLIC SAUCE

This is the Lighten Up version of the French and Spanish aïoli that tastes so wonderful on holiday. Everybody knows garlic is good for you – and it's even healthier when you eat it raw. If you're worried about the antisocial aspects of eating raw garlic, try chewing some fresh parsley after your meal.

2 plump cloves of garlic, crushed
150ml/5floz mayonnaise (you can use
reduced-fat mayonnaise if you want)
150ml/5floz low-fat live natural yoghurt (Greek-style is best)
Salt and pepper

Simply crush the garlic and mix into the mayonnaise and yoghurt, season to taste and leave covered in the fridge for at least an hour for the garlic flavour to permeate the mixture.

Serve instead of butter with crusty bread as they do in the Mediterranean. Use it as a dressing for potato or pasta salads, or serve it with grilled fish.

Variations: To this base add a peeled, stoned avocado and whiz together until smooth, using a hand-held bar blender; or make it into a bean pâté or dip by whizzing with a drained can of cannellini beans or chickpeas, sharpened with a little lemon or lime juice, and seasoned with salt and paprika pepper.

TOMATO DRESSING

A tasty, extremely low-fat way to dress green salads, slaws and pasta salads. Base it on tomato juice or the thicker tomato passata, adding just a tablespoon of olive oil to about 150ml/¼pt of passata; flavour with a little wine or balsamic vinegar, garlic, chilli, soy sauce, honey and ginger, or with wholegrain mustard, honey and black pepper.

CREAMY CUCUMBER DRESSING

You can use this instead of mayonnaise with pasta or potato salads. Spoon it over a salad of sliced avocado and tomato, or use it to top jacket potatoes or kebabs served with salad and pitta bread.

150g/5floz Greek-style thick low-fat live yoghurt
175g/6oz piece cucumber, chopped
Few sprigs fresh dill or 1 tsp dried dill
2 tsp olive oil
2–3tsp white-wine or cider vinegar, to taste
Salt and pepper

Place all the ingredients in a jug and blend with a hand-held bar blender for a few seconds until smooth. Taste and adjust the seasonings.

Variations: Replace the dill with fresh chopped mint, adding garlic to taste.

AVOCADO AND TOFU (OR BEAN) DIP

Both tofu (fermented soya bean curd) and beans are a great source of protein, which would make this dip into a well-balanced light meal needing only the addition of some vegetable crudités and bread, pitta bread or rice cakes.

1 small ripe avocado, peeled and stoned
115g/4oz silken tofu
2 tbsp low-fat quark, yoghurt or fromage frais
1 tbsp lemon juice
Salt or garlic salt and paprika pepper

Place all the ingredients in a jug and purée with a hand-held bar blender until smooth. Taste and add more seasoning if needed.

Variation: Instead of tofu use a drained can of cannellini, flageolet or butter beans or chickpeas.

DIPPERS

Vegetables:
Use vegetables instead of fatty, salty crisps or tortilla chips in these wonderful dips: whole radishes, broccoli, spring onions, cauliflower, chicory, mangetout, baby sweetcorn and carrots, courgettes and celery cut into sticks.

Poppadoms:
Put the poppadoms in the microwave for one minute each, then break them into dipping size pieces.

Pitta crisps:
Make pitta crisps by splitting pitta breads through the centre using a sharp knife, cutting them into wedges and grilling or baking them until they are crispy and golden brown, which will happen very quickly as they are so thin. A light spritz of oil from the oil-spray before grilling will give even better colour and crispness.

TABBOULEH

Tabbouleh or cracked wheat salad is easy to make and convenient to take for a packed lunch or picnic. Simply soak the cracked wheat in water, according to the instructions on the pack, then add a handful of chopped fresh parsley and mint, a crushed clove of garlic and the finely grated zest and juice of a lemon, together with finely diced spring onion, cucumber and tomato. Season it well, garnish with a few black olives and serve with hummus and pitta bread.

GREEN SALAD

A recipe for green salad? Surely we cannot be serious. Well, yes, we are. Green salad is the ultimate slimming food – especially if you stick to lettuce without any dressing at all. So we thought it was time to set the record straight and give the green salad a new lease of life.

Start with watercress and chicory, add thinly sliced spring onion, courgette, pepper, mangetout and celery, with some sprouted seeds or sea vegetables. Toss with a little herb dressing and top with a few slivers of parmesan. The addition of some sliced avocado, pale-green flageolet beans or leftover rice or pasta would turn it into a complete meal. This is great for packed lunches too.

RICH RED SALAD

The orange and red vegetables in this salad are particularly rich in the antioxidant beta carotenes, so try this dazzling combination, then make up some of your own. Mix red oak leaf lettuce and radicchio with a little sliced red onion, red pepper, tomato, radish, beetroot and fresh orange wedges; dress it with a tablespoon of olive oil, teaspoon of balsamic vinegar, salt and pepper. Make it into a complete meal by adding a little crumbled stilton or feta cheese and some red kidney beans.

These three salads would look wonderful together as part of a buffet table or barbecue party.

BEETROOT, PEAR AND PECORINO SALAD

This is a super salad, good enough to be the starter for a dinner party, or for a light lunch. On to a bed of mixed salad leaves scatter thinly sliced fresh cooked beetroot (sold in packs from the salad counter, not the pickled variety) with sliced ripe pear and a few shavings of fresh pecorino or parmesan cheese. Whizz a handful of fresh herbs in the blender with your favourite low-calorie dressing and drizzle over.

SPINACH, CHICKPEA AND FETTA SALAD WITH CREAMY LEMON YOGHURT DRESSING

This is another complete-meal salad, great for packed lunches and picnics. Simply mix together torn baby spinach leaves with a drained can of chickpeas, a small bulb of fennel or celery, finely sliced, and a little crumbled feta cheese. Scatter with a few black olives. Make a lemon yoghurt dressing to spoon over the salad by adding a tablespoon of lemon to the Garlic Sauce recipe on page 393.

AUTUMN SALAD WITH TAHINI DRESSING

Very much nicer than standard coleslaw; try a mixture of grated carrot and celeriac, with chopped celery and apple. Make a dressing with equal quantities (about 1 tablespoon each) of tahini, water, lemon juice and olive oil, seasoned with salt and pepper. Sprinkle with a few toasted sunflower or sesame seeds.

Toppings and flavourings for chicken and fish

Pieces of fish or chicken make a very simple, nutritious meal, but they can be rather boring. These flavourings can be sprinkled over each portion in a baking dish and covered with foil. Or wrap each portion up with its flavourings in a foil parcel.

Choose chicken breasts, drumsticks and/or thighs and use sharp kitchen scissors or a small knife to remove all the skin, which is where the fat is stored.

You can use any kind of fish you like – but remember that the oily fish such as mackerel, herrings and sardines are a good source of essential fatty acids as well as protein.

MEDITERRANEAN

Crushed garlic, finely grated lemon zest and finely chopped parsley mixed together and put into a liquidiser or spice grinder, or even chopped by hand Almost every Mediterranean country has its own version of this wonderfully aromatic flavouring and you can vary it by adding pine nuts or parmesan cheese. Any leftovers can be tightly covered and kept in the fridge for a couple of days, ready to sprinkle on top of other dishes.

ORIENTAL

Finely chop about a ½ inch of fresh peeled ginger. Add a crushed clove of garlic, a few chopped spring onions, a little chilli to taste and the juice of half a lime, plus a teaspoonful of both olive oil and honey to give a mellow flavour. This mixture will be enough for one portion, so just multiply it up according to how much you want.

JAPANESE STYLE

Ideal for fresh tuna, chicken or tofu. Try mixing 1–2 tablespoons of soy sauce, sake or dry sherry, and rice vinegar with a teaspoon of sugar and a tablespoon of sesame oil. When cooked, serve sprinkled with toasted sesame seeds, with Japanese noodles.

TOMATO

A can of chopped tomatoes in juice, plus garlic paste and sweet chilli sauce or Tabasco to taste, with a few black olives scattered on top.

SWEETCORN AND PEPPER

A can of creamed sweetcorn with a chopped red or yellow pepper, lots of fresh herbs and a spoonful of low-fat quark or crème fraiche on top.

MUSHROOM

Mushrooms, red pepper, garlic and spring onions all sliced together can be given a Japanese flavour by adding a little teriyaki or soy sauce.

ORANGE, GINGER AND STAR ANISE

Lovely warm flavours are ideal for fish, poultry or meat. To the juice and finely grated zest of an orange, add a tablespoon of light soy sauce, 1 teaspoon of olive oil and ½ a teaspoon of both powdered ginger and star anise or 1 teaspoon Chinese five spice powder.

SHERRY AND MUSTARD

This marinade is ideal for a nice piece of steak or small joint of beef. Simply mix 1 tablespoon wholegrain mustard with a table-spoon of sherry or wine and 1 teaspoon of oil. Rub into the meat and leave to marinate before grilling or roasting. (Enough for 1 or 2 steaks; double up for more or a larger joint of meat.)

PESTO AND CRÈME FRAICHE

Pesto has the most wonderful flavour and combines with fish really well but is rather high in calories, so enjoy all the flavour by 'stretching' it and making a creamy sauce with the addition of low-fat crème fraiche. Per portion use 1 teaspoon pesto stirred into 2 tablespoon low-fat crème fraiche or fromage frais. Spread on to a portion of fish or skinless chicken breast and wrap in tin-foil before baking.

APPLE, TARRAGON AND MUSTARD

Mix 2 tablespoons of fresh apple juice with 1 teaspoon of cider vinegar, 1–2 tablespoons fresh chopped tarragon and 1–2 teaspoons of Dijon mustard. This particularly suits lean pork fillet with the addition of sliced onion and apple all wrapped in a tin-foil parcel.

Sauces and toppings for pasta, rice, polenta and potatoes

★ Chopped smoked salmon scraps, low-fat soft cheese or fromage frais, lemon juice and dried or fresh dill
★ Prawns, diced cucumber, fromage frais, lemon juice and mayonnaise
★ Tomato passata, broccoli, courgettes and parmesan
★ Bacon or tofu, peas or sweetcorn with fromage frais, yoghurt or soft cheese
★ A can of cannellini or flageolet beans, tuna, tomato, red pepper and olives
★ Marinated or smoked tofu or chicken stir-fried with a pack of fresh or frozen stir-fry vegetables and sweet chilli sauce
★ Cottage cheese with a little curry powder, a few raisins or fresh grapes and toasted pine nuts

★ Tuna mixed with a drained can of mixed beans and sweet chilli sauce
★ Wilted spinach with poached egg

Leftovers

Leftovers sound like second best – but leftovers from simple, good-quality meals are a lot better for you than a takeaway kebab, which is often the kind of alternative that springs to mind. Leftovers don't have to be tired, dried up or curling at the edges – they are positive forward planning and you can use them in salads, picnics and packed lunches as well as snack suppers. You could spend the time you've saved in meal preparation on some extra Fat Jar or Feel Good Fitness exercise.

★ Cook extra rice to use in rice salad. Add peas, sweetcorn or a drained can of flageolet beans with cooked chicken, canned tuna or a few toasted sunflower seeds. Season with lots of fresh herbs, Tabasco if you like a little heat, or lime or lemon juice. Be careful with rice, though – it's notorious for causing stomach upsets if it's left sitting around at room temperature. Don't keep it for more than a day, and refrigerate it as soon as it's cooled enough after cooking.
★ New potatoes can be added to garlic dressing with other vegetables like diced tomatoes, cucumber, crunchy celery and olives. Almost anything tastes good like this.
★ Mashed potato can be turned into fish cakes with fresh or frozen cod, haddock or salmon, or canned mackerel or tuna. Shape them on a floured board and cook in a non-stick frying pan with a spritz of oil.
★ Cook extra pasta, then after draining it, refresh the leftover portion in cold water to cool it before draining again, this will stop it overcooking in its own heat and sticking together. For an Oriental flavour add finely shredded carrot, spring onion, celery and courgette, and a dressing of rice vinegar, soy sauce, ginger and a little honey. Mix in leftover cooked chicken, fish or shellfish or canned tuna.
★ Quorn and rice salad can be made very quickly out of left-over white or brown rice with an equal quantity of Quorn or

marinated tofu chunks. Add a few cooked peas or some sweetcorn, a chopped red or yellow pepper and a few seedless grapes or chopped apple. Make a dressing of 2 teaspoons of sesame oil, 2 teaspoons of Chinese rice vinegar, a little grated fresh ginger and a good sprinkle of toasted sesame and sunflower seeds to garnish.

Box lunches and sandwich fillings

PROSCIUTTO-WRAPPED CHICKEN

Prosciutto (Parma ham) or the Spanish Serrano is extremely low-fat and has such a rich, concentrated flavour that you need less. Simply wrap strips of the ham round fingers of cold leftover chicken or goat's cheese. Pack on a bed of salad made from lettuce or spinach leaves, with thinly sliced courgette, red peppers, celery or fennel and baby tomatoes. Take a little dressing or a wedge of lemon to dress the salad just before eating.

CREAMY PASTA SALAD

Use leftover cooked pasta to make a quick salad. Toss the pasta with Garlic Sauce (see page 393) and add leftover cooked chicken, salmon etc., raw, sliced button mushrooms, tiny florets of broccoli and baby tomatoes.

CARROT AND CUMIN SOUP

Cook an onion with carrots in vegetable stock flavoured with a little ground cumin. Liquidise until smooth, pack in a flask and take pitta breads split open and spread with low-fat soft cheese and alfalfa sprouts or watercress.

SANDWICH FILLINGS

★ Tuna, sundried tomato paste and spring onion
★ Cottage cheese and kiwi fruit or strawberries with black pepper

- ★ Peanut butter with alfalfa sprouts
- ★ Hummus with grated carrot and sliced cucumber
- ★ Tuna, sweetcorn, low-fat fromage frais and a pinch of curry powder
- ★ Smoked tofu, tomato chutney and watercress
- ★ Leftover char-grilled or roast vegetables with slivers of fresh parmesan or goat's cheese
- ★ To make your own low-fat cheese, simply tip a pot of low-fat live yoghurt into a fine sieve or sieve lined with a piece of muslin and leave over a bowl to drain until you have a soft-cheese consistency. Use this as a spread on bread instead of butter or margarine.
- ★ For a sweet snack, with a cheesecake flavour, drain a pot of fruit yogurt as above and spread on to rye bread or a cracker, and top with sliced banana, strawberry etc. Tastes great and very indulgent but it's not.
- ★ Low-fat soft cheese, avocado and tomato
- ★ Soft cheese, marmite and sliced tomato
- ★ Soft cheese, smoked salmon, chives and a squeeze of lemon

ITALIAN MIXED BEAN AND BASIL BAGUETTE

Serves 2

200g/7oz tin of mixed Italian beans
1 tsp passata
1 tsp garlic purée
8 fresh basil leaves
½ tsp extra virgin olive oil
1 baguette
Mixed salad leaves

Put the beans, passata, garlic purée, basil and olive oil into a liquidiser and blend into a fairly smooth paste.

Spread the paste inside the baguette and then fill with the salad leaves.

Dynamic snacks

When you're caught out by hunger pangs (real ones that register higher than 6 on the Hunger Scale), there's no need to resort to the Coke and Mars bar solution. They will only make you feel hungry again soon afterwards because of the insulin rush that will follow the sugar hit – and just think of the empty calories.

Always be prepared. Keep some of these in your bag or your car, or your desk, so that you don't get desperate and do something you'll regret later.

★ Fresh fruit is probably the best. It's sweet, but it has a lot of nutritional value. Just don't let it get so ripe that the sugar is absorbed too fast. Bananas and satsumas are the easiest because they are ready packaged, but you can wash grapes and other fruit at home and keep them in a box. Always wash your fruit – especially if it isn't organic. The government is even issuing warnings about pesticides now.

★ Dried fruit is great but bag it up into small portions so you don't get carried away and eat too much. Even natural fruit sugars can still cause a blood sugar 'high' in some people if they eat a lot of it. Try a mixture of apricots, dates, raisins, dried banana slices, pineapple, papaya, but make sure they are natural and not sugar-coated.

★ Dried fruit bars, sometimes known as fruit 'leather' are available from health food stores. They are simply unsweetened fruit purées, dried and pressed into a thin sheet.

★ Some muesli bars are OK, but most of them have a lot of added sugar (usually in several different forms) so at least read the labels. Sugar is often the main ingredient in these 'healthy' snacks.

★ Nuts and seeds are natural and good for you as long as you don't eat too many. You could make your own mixture of sunflower seeds, sesame seeds, pine nuts, cashew nuts etc. Dry roast them in a non-stick pan over a medium heat but you have to stir or shake the pan almost constantly to allow them to brown evenly. Tip them out into a bowl and add a drizzle of soy sauce. Stir to coat them evenly and leave to cool.

★ Marmite-flavoured rice cakes make a savoury alternative to crisps.

★ Home-made popcorn is easy to make either in a large pan with a lid or in special microwave packs. Sprinkle over a little salt and/or chilli, or serve sweet with a little cinnamon and some dried fruit.

★ Make apple or pear 'crisps' by slicing the fruit as thinly as possible with a mandolin, then spread them out in a single layer on greaseproof or non-stick paper and dry them out in the oven until they just start to brown.

★ Home-made oven chips are amazingly good and virtually fat free. One kilo (2lb 4oz) of potatoes cut into chunky chips need only 1 tablespoon oil (or a few spritzes with an oil spray) to toss them in before spreading out on a baking sheet and baking in a hot oven for about 30 minutes. Season with salt and pepper, or toss in some herbs or spices before baking.

★ Corn on the cob makes a great snack to keep you going and it doesn't really need to be dripping in butter. A quick spritz of the oil spray makes it look tempting enough. Just simmer them gently in boiling water, or steam, or even wrap in foil and oven-roast as they do on the streets in the Eastern Mediterranean.

Desserts

The perfect pudding is a small and delicate work of art. By the time you get to the pudding you've probably already eaten all the food you really need, so consider it as more of a visual treat than anything else.

You can make some lovely, simple puddings with fruit and very little sugar or fat.

★ Baked apples with sultanas
★ Poached pears with a little orange juice and flaked almonds
★ Stewed fruit with cinnamon and nutmeg, served with low-fat yoghurt
★ Stewed fruit with muesli or oat topping
★ Baked banana with a little honey, lemon and cinnamon (great on the barbecue)

* Winter fruit salad: dried fruit soaked with spices and served hot
* Summer fruit salads that are colour co-ordinated and beautifully arranged

MIXED SUMMER BERRIES WITH
RASPBERRY SAUCE AND RICOTTA CHEESE

Serves 2

300g/11oz mixed summer berries (strawberries, blackberries, blueberries, raspberries)
85g/3oz ricotta cheese
½ tablespoon clear honey
25g/1oz flaked almonds

Sauce:
100g/3½oz raspberries
1 tablespoon fresh orange juice

Wash the berries and leave to dry.

Make the sauce by puréeing the raspberries in the food processor/liquidiser and sieving them to remove the pips. Mix the raspberry purée with the orange juice.

Beat together the ricotta and the honey.

Arrange the berries on a large plate and serve with a dollop of the ricotta and honey, sprinkle with the almonds and finally pour over the raspberry sauce.

Dinner party menus

FIRST MENU

AVOCADO AND GARLIC SAUCE
WITH CRUDITÉS AND PITTA CRISPS

Using the recipe for Garlic Sauce on page 393, add an avocado to this delicious mixture to make a dip. Spoon into individual small dishes (tiny soufflé dishes or ramekins would be ideal) and place one on each serving plate.

Prepare lots of fresh vegetable crudités and arrange round, together with pitta crisps – see page 395.

Alternatively use the recipe for Avocado and Tofu Dip on page 395.

SALMON TERIYAKI

Serves 4
Cooking time: 5 minutes

4 salmon fillets
1 tbsp olive oil
2 tbsp teriyaki sauce
1 tbsp clear honey
Juice and zest of 1 lime
Wedges of lime to garnish

Line the grill pan with tinfoil and lay on the salmon fillets.

Mix together the oil, teriyaki sauce, honey and lime juice and zest. Pour this over the salmon, turning the fish to coat both sides. Leave to marinate for at least 20 minutes.

Heat the grill, then cook the salmon for 4–5 minutes, turning once and spooning over the marinade.

Serve with the juices poured over, garnished with lime wedges, with sugar snaps and tiny new potatoes or saffron mash.

GRILLED CARAMELISED PINEAPPLE
WITH PASSION FRUIT COULIS

Sprinkle slices of fresh pineapple with a tablespoon of soft brown sugar and grill under a preheated grill until melted and caramelised. Put one slice on to each serving plate.

Halve one passion fruit per person and scoop out the flesh. Stir in little Kirsch or white rum to flavour and spoon around the pineapple.

Garnish with a sprig of fresh mint and serve with honeyed plain yoghurt or low-fat fromage frais.

SMOKED SALMON AND DILL PÂTÉ

Serves 4

150g/5½oz smoked salmon pieces
200g/7oz low-fat soft cheese
juice of 1 lemon
2 tbsp roughly chopped fresh dill (reserve 4 sprigs)

Place the smoked salmon, soft cheese and lemon juice into a food processor and blitz to form a smooth mixture. Remove the blade and stir in the dill. Scrape out into a bowl. If the mixture is too stiff, add a little plain yoghurt to achieve the right consistency.

Heap the mixture on to thin slices of toasted baguette and garnish with sprigs of fresh dill.

LOUISIANA BLACKENED CHICKEN

There's nothing boring about this chicken dish – the flavours explode on the palate. It can also be made with turkey breast fillets and is great served cold for picnics.

Serves 4
Cooking time: 12–15 minutes

4 boneless, skinless chicken breasts
½tsp salt
½tsp gound black pepper
½tsp paprika pepper
½tsp garlic powder
½tsp dried oregano
½tsp dried thyme
2 tbsp oil

Preheat the oven to 200C/400F/Gas Mark 6.

Cut each chicken breast into 3 long strips. In a large bowl mix together all the dry seasonings and toss in the chicken strips (toss very well to make sure each one is evenly coated).

Heat the oil in a large frying pan and fry the chicken pieces on both sides over high heat just to seal the chicken and roast the spices.

Transfer the chicken to a roasting tin and continue cooking in the oven for 10–12 minutes until the chicken is cooked through.

Serve the chicken with rice and wilted spinach with Garlic Sauce (see page 393).

APRICOT YOGHURT ICE

A simple ice-cream maker is ideal if you like ice-creams and sorbets, as it enables you to make your own low-fat, additive-free, healthy desserts. Complicated recipes just aren't necessary, the simplest are usually the best.

Soak, then cook 225g/8oz dried apricots in enough water just to cover. Sweeten to taste and add a few drops of natural vanilla extract. Cool, then purée the mixture with a bar blender or in the liquidiser. Add a large pot of low-fat Greek yoghurt and whizz again. Taste to check for sweetness, then pour into an ice-cream maker or polythene freezer box. Freeze until needed. To serve, spoon into small glasses and if liked pour over a little Amaretti or Kirsch and serve with Amaretti biscuits.

THIRD MENU

PROSCIUTTO AND PEAR SALAD IN RADICCHIO

Carefully remove each whole leaf from the radicchio and wash gently. Place one large or two small leaves on to each serving plate. Shred the remaining leaves and place in a mixing bowl.

Cut a 70g/2oz pack of Prosciutto ham into thin strips and add to the bowl, together with one large or two small ripe pears, chopped, and a handful of torn basil leaves. Mix together and spoon into the radicchio leaves.

Make the dressing by mixing together 4 tablespoons of plain yoghurt with 2 tablespoons of water and 1 tablespoon of pesto.

Season and spoon over and around each serving; garnish with more basil leaves.

Serve with chunks of warm ciabatta bread.

TIGER PRAWN PROVENÇAL

Serves 4
Cooking time: 6 minutes

1 tbsp olive oil
2 cloves garlic, crushed
1 small red chilli, finely chopped or 1–2 tbsp sweet chilli sauce
400g/14oz raw tiger prawns, peeled
1 large ripe beefsteak tomato, skinned and finely chopped
4 sundried tomatoes in oil, drained and chopped
1 tbsp white-wine vinegar or lemon juice
8 pitted black olives, halved
Salt and black pepper
Fresh basil leaves

Heat the oil in a frying pan or wok and add the garlic and fresh chilli. Fry gently for a minute to soften but not brown, then add the prawns and stir-fry over a medium-to-high heat for 2–3 minutes until the prawns have turned pink.

Add the chopped tomato and sundried tomatoes, vinegar and olives, and cook for a further 2 minutes. Season and add a few torn basil leaves.

Serve immediately, with rice scattered with more torn basil leaves.

RASPBERRY AND ELDERFLOWER FOOL

Serves 4

200g/7oz raspberries
400g/14oz Low-fat Greek yoghurt or fromage frais
4 tbsp elderflower cordial

A delectable and incredibly easy dessert: simply mash or purée the fresh raspberries and fold into the low-fat Greek yogurt or fromage frais and sweeten with the elderflower cordial. Spoon into small dishes or glasses and top with a sprig of fresh mint or lemon balm.

FOURTH MENU

WARM SPINACH SALAD

Serves 4
Cooking Time : 2–3 minutes

1 tbsp olive oil
1 red onion, thinly sliced
1 clove garlic, crushed
2 tbsp pine nuts
6 sundried tomatoes in oil, drained and cut into strips
2 tbsp balsamic vinegar
225g/8oz bag baby spinach
Handful fresh basil leaves
piece fresh parmesan, flaked

Heat the oil in a frying pan or wok and add the sliced onion, garlic and pine nuts. Cook over fairly high heat until the nuts begin to brown. Add the sundried tomatoes.

Add the balsamic vinegar, remove from the heat and mix thoroughly. Add the spinach and basil and toss well. Pile on to each serving plate and sprinkle with a few flakes of fresh parmesan. Serve with warm crusty bread.

The Catalan Spanish have a variation of this dish adding a few raisins instead of the sundried tomatoes and replacing the pine nuts with flaked almonds.

PORK STEAKS WITH
WILD MUSHROOM SAUCE

Serves 4
Cooking time: 15 minutes

4 pork shoulder steaks
1 tbsp oil
2 cloves garlic, crushed
280g/10oz mushrooms, sliced
1 tbsp tomato purée
1 tbsp redcurrant jelly
½–1tsp sweet paprika pepper and a little salt
150ml/¼pt beef stock
150ml/¼pt red wine or stock
1 tbsp cornflour

Trim any excess fat from the pork. Heat a non-stick frying pan and give it a light spritz of oil. Seal the pork on both sides, then reduce the heat to medium and cook for 3–4 minutes on both sides or until cooked through. Remove from the pan and keep warm.

To make the sauce add the oil to the pan, then the garlic and mushrooms and cook, stirring frequently, for 2–3 minutes. Add the tomato purée, redcurrant jelly, and the paprika and salt. Stir to mix, then add the stock and red wine. Mix the cornflour with a little water and stir into the sauce, bring to the boil and simmer for a few minutes.

Return the pork to the pan to heat. Serve with rice, new potatoes or polenta and lots of vegetables.

SPICE ISLAND BANANAS

In a large non-stick frying pan melt 25g/1oz of butter and add 2 tablespoons of soft brown sugar.

Add the juice and finely grated rind of an orange and 1 teaspoon of cinnamon. Bubble together before adding 4 large quartered bananas.

Cook together for 2–3 minutes, then pour in a good slug of rum or Tia Maria, or whatever you have.

Serve immediately with a low-fat ice-cream or tropical fruit sorbet.

FIFTH MENU

THYME AND PARMESAN POLENTA WITH BALSAMIC MUSHROOMS

A very easy starter that can be prepared in advance. Make instant polenta according to the packet instructions using vegetable stock and fresh thyme to flavour. Pour into a flat square cake tin. Dust with grated parmesan and allow to cool. Cut into triangles and grill or griddle just before serving. Top with sliced mushrooms cooked in a little olive oil and flavoured with a little balsamic vinegar. Garnish with a few flakes of parmesan and fresh thyme or parsley.

ROASTED VEGETABLE COUSCOUS

Serves 4
Cooking time: 30-40 minutes

2 large parsnips, peeled
2 sticks celery or 1 bulb fennel
2 sweet potatoes, peeled
1 large red onion
2 large courgettes
1 large red pepper, deseeded
8–12 whole unpeeled cloves garlic
2 tbsp olive oil
Few sprigs fresh rosemary and thyme
350g/12oz couscous
1 tsp cayenne pepper and a little salt
Juice of 1 lemon
Chopped fresh coriander

Preheat the oven to 200C/400F/Gas Mark 6.

Cut the parsnips and celery (or fennel) into chunks and cook in boiling salted water for 2–3 minutes, then drain and tip into a greased large roasting tin. Add the sweet potato, onion, courgettes and red pepper all cut into large chunks. Sprinkle over the garlic cloves, then drizzle over the oil. Toss the vegetables in the oil to coat evenly, strew the herbs over the top and roast in the oven for 30–40 minutes or until golden brown.

Cook the couscous according to packet instructions, then season with the cayenne pepper and salt and lemon juice.

Serve the couscous on a large dish with the roasted vegetables over the top, sprinkled with the coriander.

There are so many variations to this theme: use your own favourite vegetables – pumpkin and squash are ideal when in season, chickpeas or other beans can be added to make the dish even more substantial, raisins and pine nuts can be added to the couscous for extra flavour.

WATERMELON WITH LIME, MINT AND GINGER SYRUP

Serves 4

4 generous slices watermelon
1 tbsp clear honey
2 tbsp shredded fresh mint
2 chunks of ginger preserved in syrup

This wonderfully fresh-tasting dessert can be made ahead of time, covered tightly with cling film and refrigerated. If watermelon is not in season, use any other melon or combination of varieties and colours.

Cut the melon into chunky cubes and put into a bowl. Add the honey and mint. Cut the ginger into very thin strips and add to the bowl, together with a tablespoon of the syrup. Gently mix everything together and leave for the flavours to mingle for at least an hour.

THE JOYS OF EATING

You may be surprised at some of the ingredients in these recipes: sugar, eggs and rum, for example – is this really a slimming book?

We aren't suggesting that you eat lots of these ingredients or that you eat them often. A little of any of them goes a long way and a teaspoon of sugar, for instance, can be quite enough to bring out the flavour of a dessert or a dressing.

If you always check the Hunger Scale and run the Think Before You Eat exercise you won't be in danger of eating too much of anything. Another good way to make sure you're eating only what you need is to concentrate on enjoying your food. Slow down your eating, make a meal of it, really taste all the ingredients and smell every mouthful before you eat it. In fact, if you happen to be doing the cooking you can also concentrate on choosing all the best ingredients.

Cooking and eating are two of life's great pleasures – so enjoy!

ACKNOWLEDGEMENTS

The following experts have contributed to this book. We are especially grateful to Justin Roberts for the nutritional guidelines in Chapter 17 and to Colin Deans for all the detailed information about how to start your own exercise programme in Chapter 18.

Justin Roberts, MPhil, DipION, ACSM
BASES Accredited Sport and Exercise Physiologist
Member of the British Association of Nutritional Therapy

Colin Deans
Head of Training at Premier Training and Development

Anne Gains
Consultant Home Economist, Food and Nutrition Writer

Caroline Harper, PhD
Brain chemistry consultant

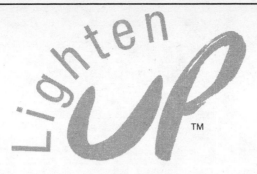

A range of Lighten Up courses and products are now available. To receive your **free information pack**

call us on **0845 603 3456**
(calls charged at local rate)

visit us at **www.lightenup.co.uk**

email us at **info@lightenup.co.uk**

or return the slip below to

Lighten Up Ltd
46 Staines Road Twickenham TW2 5AH

PLEASE SEND A FREE INFORMATION PACK TO:

Title: First name: Surname:

Address:

            Postcode:

Home phone:

email address: